S0-AGM-021

Anxiety & Stress
Self Help Book

Dr. Susan Lark's

Anxiety & Stress
Self Help Book

Susan Lark, M.D.

*Effective solutions for nervous tension,
emotional distress, anxiety, and panic*

CELESTIALARTS

Berkeley, California

*To my wonderful husband Jim and
my darling daughter Rebecca.
To the health and well-being of all women.*

NOTE: The information in this book is meant to complement the advice and guidance of your physician, not replace it. It is very important that women with any symptoms of anxiety or stress be evaluated by a physician. If you are under the care of a physician, you should discuss any major changes in your regimen with him or her. Because this is a book and not a medical consultation, keep in mind that the information presented here may not apply in your particular case. Whenever a question arises, discuss it with your physician.

Copyright 1993, 1996 by Dr. Susan Lark. All rights reserved.
No part of this book may be reproduced in any form, except for brief review, without the written permission of the publisher.

CELESTIAL ARTS
P.O. Box 7123, Berkeley, CA 94707

Cover design by Fifth Street Design
Text design and composition by Brad Greene
Photographs by Ronald May
Illustrations by Shelley Reeves Smith

Library of Congress Cataloging-in-Publication Data
Lark, Susan M., 1945-
    Dr. Susan Lark's anxiety & stress self help book : effective solutions for
nervous tension, emotional distress, anxiety, & panic / Susan Lark.
        p.   cm.
    Includes bibliographical references and index.
    ISBN 0-89087-775-0
    1. Anxiety. 2. Stress (Psychology).   3. Stress management.   4. Women-
-Psychology.   I. Title.
BF575.A6L35 1996
152.4'6--dc20
                                                                    95-37723
                                                                    CIP

Contents

Introduction

A Self Help Approach to Anxiety and Stress

Emotional symptoms due to excessive life stresses are very common in our society and affect many millions of women. Upset feelings created by stress can trigger nervous tension, irritability, and edginess. In extreme cases, women will react to stress with feelings of anxiety. In fact, 10 percent of the American population—between 20 million and 30 million people—suffer from anxiety symptoms each year. These numbers are astonishing, especially since the symptoms of emotional distress are not limited to a particular age group. Rather, anxiety symptoms occur in women of all ages, from preadolescence to the postmenopausal years.

When anxiety feelings are excessive, they can express themselves in episodes of fear and panic. They may even trigger unpleasant physical symptoms such as rapid heart beat and shortness of breath, leaving a woman's physical body feeling as upset and out of control as her emotions. Anxiety can impede a woman's ability to function optimally in the workplace, at home, and with co-workers, friends, and family.

Emotional symptoms such as anxiety stem from a broad range of emotional, social, chemical, and physical imbalances. Some women have anxiety episodes that are emotionally based in childhood upsets and traumas, while others may develop stress symptoms after severe life crises such as a death, divorce, or job loss. Anxiety can also be a primary symptom of medical problems such as PMS, transition into menopause, hyperthyroidism, and hypoglycemia, as well as other health-related issues. And, anxiety can arise from nutritional deficiencies as well as the improper use of drugs or alcohol.

Historically, women with anxiety have been treated with drug therapies, sometimes combined with counseling or psychotherapy. Though antianxiety drugs help relieve the emotional symptoms, they can be a mixed blessing for many women. Often they produce unpleasant side effects as well as psychological and physical dependence. Counseling may be ineffective if underlying physical causes of anxiety are not diagnosed or are ignored. Many women have told me of their fruitless search for adequate relief as they went from physician to physician, trying different combinations of medications.

What is missing from this scenario is the woman's participation in her own healing process. In my experience, women can reap tremendous benefits from learning and practicing anxiety-relieving self help techniques. These techniques, which encompass specific principles of diet, nutrition, exercise, and stress management, can often replace medication as a treatment. Even in more severe cases of anxiety, the use of self help techniques along with medication produces better results for the patient than medication alone. In addition, the practice of self help techniques can assist women to reduce not only their dependence on medication, but also the likelihood of the debilitating anxiety symptoms recurring.

Learning to Help My Patients

Over the past 20 years, many of my patients who suffered from anxiety and other stress-related emotional symptoms have greatly benefited from self-care programs. I have spent years researching the use of diet, nutrition, and many other lifestyle techniques as part of a complete approach to treating these problems. Specific acupressure points, yoga stretches, and exercise routines, as well as many other stress management techniques offer a wide variety of self-care options. My goal with patients has always been to provide the information, education, and resources to help them relieve their symptoms by becoming healthier women and then maintain this state through healthy lifestyle practices. I have been delighted with the positive feedback that my patients give me. They are always pleased and relieved to find that self help treatments are so beneficial and effective.

How to Use This Book

My purpose for writing this book is to share with women the self-care techniques that I have found through many years of medical practice to be most useful. I practice these techniques, too. Preventive health care has had tremendous benefits for me; I am healthier and more productive now than ten years ago. I plan to feel better and to be even healthier ten years from now. Expanding my knowledge about self help and continually researching new health-care techniques for treating anxiety is a major goal in my practice.

The anxiety and stress self help program provides important information for all women suffering from these problems. The program is written so that each woman reading this book can select from a wide variety of self help treatment options. A treatment plan that utilizes only one method and purports to be the only treatment for these two problems will probably work for only a small percentage of women. In my medical practice, I have better results when I individualize each patient's treatment program. By overlapping treatments from various disciplines, most women find combinations that work for them. You will be able to find a combination that works for you, too.

This program is set up to enable you to develop your own treatment plan. All the methods you need are contained in this book. They include information on diet and nutrition, as well as material on vitamins, minerals, and herbs that, over the past two decades, I have found to be effective for anxiety and stress symptom relief. Nutritional supplementation is an important part of an optimal health program for women with anxiety and stress. Programs of stress reduction, physical exercise, acupressure massage, deep breathing exercises, and yoga that are specifically helpful for anxiety and stress are also important parts of this book. A chapter on drug therapies is included so that you can be fully informed about the most effective medical treatments.

Read through the entire book first to familiarize yourself with the material. The Anxiety Workbook (chapter 2) will help you evaluate your symptoms, risk factors, and stress-creating lifestyle habits. Then turn to the therapy chapters and read through the rest of the book. Try all the therapies that pertain to your symptoms; some will probably make you feel better than others. Establish a regimen that works for you and use it every day.

This anxiety and stress self help program is practical and easy to follow. You may use it by itself or in conjunction with a medical program. Though working with a physician or psychologist may be necessary to establish a definitive diagnosis of the cause of anxiety, and medical therapy may still be necessary if you have moderate to severe symptoms, do not underestimate the importance of a good self help program. For many women, this book can help speed up the diagnostic process. My self help techniques can play a major role in reducing the severity of your symptoms and preventing recurrence of the disease process. With a self-help program, you can experience a feeling of wellness that will radiate out and touch your whole life. You will have more time and energy to enjoy your work, family, and other pleasures in life. Just like my patients, you may positively transform your life by following these beneficial self help techniques.

Identifying
the Problem

1

What Is Anxiety?

The word *anxiety* means "a state of being uneasy, apprehensive, or worried about what may happen." It is also described as a "feeling of being powerless and unable to cope with threatening events . . . [characterized] by physical tension." Though this is a dictionary definition, it certainly fits the way that many women feel about their lives today. The frequency with which women feel anxiety is reflected in my medical practice: My patients complain about anxiety and other emotional symptoms more than anything else. This is true whether they are seeking help for primarily psychological or physical ailments.

The Emotions of Anxiety

Anxiety for most of us is an inevitable part of life. We all encounter everyday, real-life situations to which anxiety is a reasonable response. These situations can be as major as a death, divorce, or job loss, or as seemingly minor as going to the doctor or meeting new people at a social event.

Although anxiety is a very common emotional response, its expression can take different forms. It varies in intensity from being an appropriate response to stressful or difficult situations to being an actual psychiatric disorder. Disorders can occur when symptoms persist or are severe in nature. Some women have anxiety symptoms so intense that the symptoms interfere with their ability to function on a day-to-day basis.

The Physiology of Anxiety

While most women experience anxiety emotionally as upset and distress, we also react to these upsetting feelings on a physical level. What actually happens to our body when we are feeling anxious, nervous, or even panicky? Anxiety feelings normally set off an alarm reaction in our body called the "fight-or-flight" response. This response occurs to any perceived threat, whether it is physically real, psychologically upsetting, or even imaginary. Our thoughts and feelings can trigger this response; it can even occur simply when we're excited. The fight-or-flight response is a powerful protective mechanism that allows our body to mobilize energy quickly and either escape from or confront any type of danger.

The fight-or-flight response begins in our nervous system. The nervous system consists of the brain, the spinal cord, and the peripheral nerves. It is divided by function into two parts: the voluntary nervous system and the involuntary (or autonomic) nervous system.

The voluntary nervous system manages activity in the conscious domain. For example, if you place your hand on a hot stove, pain fibers will trigger a response that is sent to the brain. The brain sends back an immediate response telling you to move your hand before you burn yourself. You then pull your hand away, fast.

The autonomic nervous system regulates functions of which the average person is usually unaware, such as muscle tension, pulse rate, respiration, glandular function, and the circulation of the blood. The autonomic nervous system is also divided into two parts that oppose and complement each other: the sympathetic and parasympathetic nervous systems. These control the upper and lower limits of your physiology, respectively. For example, if excitement speeds up the heart rate too much, the parasympathetic nervous system's job is to act as a control circuit and slow it down. If the heart slows down too much, then the sympathetic nervous system's job is to speed it up.

A fight-or-flight response stimulates the sympathetic nervous system, triggering several different physical responses. Our adrenal glands increase their output of adrenaline and cortisone as body chemistry adjusts to meet the crisis. The outpouring of these hormones causes the heart and pulse rate to speed up, the breathing to become shallow and rapid, and the hands and feet to become icy cold. In addition, muscles tighten up and become tense and contracted. The sympathetic nervous system also triggers the release of stored sugar in the liver, an increase in the metabolic rate of the body, inhibition of digestion, and an excess secretion of acid in the stomach—all in response to feelings of anxiety and stress.

Though the physiological response to anxiety or stress is the same no matter what the initial stressor is (physical danger, psychological distress, or imaginary threat), the chemical trigger for anxiety can vary greatly. For example, the chemical imbalance that triggers PMS-related anxiety is often quite different from the chemical or hormonal imbalances seen in hyperthyroidism or menopause-related anxiety. I will discuss the chemical triggers as I explore the common causes of anxiety.

In women with anxiety or panic episodes, the sympathetic nervous system is actually too sensitive or too easily triggered. Their systems are too often in a state of readiness to react to a crisis. This puts them in a constant state of tension—fight-or-flight.

The Common Causes of Anxiety

When a woman identifies anxiety as a serious complaint, any of four body systems may be compromised:

- The nervous system, which comprises the fibers that connect the brain, organs, and muscles by transmitting impulses that allow normal bodily sensation and movement, as well as the experience and expression of moods and feelings.

- The endocrine or glandular system, which regulates reproductive and metabolic functions, such as menstruation and the efficient burning of food for energy. The endocrine glands communicate with one another by secreting into the bloodstream chemicals called hormones that carry chemical messages from one gland to another.

- The immune system, which fights foreign invaders in the body, such as bacteria, viruses, and cancer cells.

- The cardiovascular system, which consists of the heart and all the blood vessels in the body.

The remainder of this chapter discusses the most common physical and psychological problems in these systems that I have encountered over the years in my medical practice. Many (but not all) of them are problems often seen by any physician practicing primary care medicine. Most likely your symptoms of anxiety are related to one or more of these health problems.

Types of Anxiety Disorders

Three major types of psychologically-based anxiety disorders are most pertinent to women: generalized anxiety disorder, panic disorder, and phobias. Research in brain chemistry has shown that these anxiety disorders may also be linked to specific chemical changes in the brain, thus suggesting a strong mind-body link. The field of psychiatry recognizes other types of anxiety disorders, such as obsessive-compulsive disorder and post-traumatic stress syndrome, which I will not cover in this book; although they are important problems, they have less relevance for most women. While there tends to be some overlap in the symptoms experienced by women with the various types of anxiety disorders, there are still significant differences among the specific types.

Generalized Anxiety Disorder

Generalized anxiety disorder is characterized by chronic anxiety that tends to focus on real-life issues, such as problems with work, finances, relationships, or health, which feel dangerous or threatening to a woman's security and well-being. The emotional and physical symptoms of anxiety that these situations elicit must persist for at least six months to establish this diagnosis. Often, the real-life issues in turn elicit deeper emotional concerns, such as fear of abandonment, rejection, or not being loved. These deep fears may underlie the anxiety around troubled personal relationships, fear of failure, inability to cope effectively with stressful situations, and even fear of death when there are health concerns. Since the symptoms are experienced frequently, they can interfere with a woman's quality of life and her ability to function optimally on a daily basis.

Common symptoms include frequent upset, worry, and nervous tension, as well as insomnia, irritability, difficulty concentrating, and startling easily. Physical symptoms include the typical fight-or-flight response of rapid heartbeat, cold hands and feet, shortness of breath, muscle tension, shakiness, depression, and chronic fatigue. The symptoms, however, are not so severe as to be complicated by panic attacks and phobias. Generalized anxiety disorder can date back as early as childhood, but a majority of patients are initially diagnosed in their twenties or thirties. The disorder seems to occur with equal frequency among both men and women.

Consult a physician if you suffer from an apparent generalized anxiety disorder to rule out any possible medical disorders that could be causing these symptoms. For example, hyperthyroidism, food allergies, or PMS are often mistaken for an anxiety disorder. In addition, since anxiety and depression can coexist, it is important to know which is the primary component, as treatment can differ depending on which is primary and which is secondary.

Panic Disorder

The experience of panic is characterized by the sudden onset of intense fear or apprehension that occurs unexpectedly for no apparent reason. Usually the panic symptoms appear without prior warning, catching a person unaware; a woman is often in the middle of a panic episode before she even has time to register what is happening. Luckily, the acute phase of the panic attack tends to be short-lived, lasting only a few minutes. However, the symptoms may persist beyond the initial attack, though at a level of lesser intensity. To have the diagnosis of panic disorder, a woman must have experienced at least four panic attacks in a one-month period, or have experienced significant apprehension and worry throughout an entire month following a single panic attack. As in generalized anxiety disorder, the symptoms are typical of the fight-or-flight reaction, although panic attacks tend to be much more intense and disabling.

Since panic attacks are acute and short-lived, they also differ in duration from generalized anxiety disorder, where the symptoms are persistent and chronic. Typical symptoms include at least four of the following: rapid heartbeat or heart palpitations, chest pain, shakiness, dizziness, faintness, shortness of breath, cold hands and feet, numbness and tingling in the hands and feet, intestinal distress, sweating, feelings of losing control, and feelings of unreality. Between panic episodes, women can suffer much fear and apprehension, worrying about their recurrence. Panic disorder tends to coexist with agoraphobia (fear of open spaces or public places), which is also discussed in this chapter. In fact, panic attacks in combination with agoraphobia affect 5 percent of the population in this country, while only 1 percent suffer from panic disorder alone. Panic disorder tends to develop during the twenties in susceptible women.

It is important to differentiate panic disorder from medical problems such as mitral valve prolapse (which can coexist with panic disorder and produce similar symptoms) and hypoglycemia, or even chemical imbalances like drug withdrawal or excessive caffeine intake. A careful diagnostic evaluation should be done by a physician to make sure that a medical problem necessitating specific, nonpsychiatric therapies has not been overlooked or misdiagnosed.

Phobias

Phobias are characterized by an excessive, persistent, and often irrational fear of a person, object, place, or situation. In severe cases, the person suffering from a particular phobia will try to avoid the inciting trigger. At the very least, a phobia can create severe emotional distress and can cause a person to postpone facing situations that trigger the phobia. Day-to-day functioning or even one's health and well-being can be compromised, particularly when the phobia centers on being in public places, going to social gatherings, giving public speeches, or even seeing a doctor or dentist.

As mentioned earlier, agoraphobia (fear of open or public spaces) is fairly prevalent in our society, affecting 5 percent of the population to some degree. In fact, it is the most common of all the anxiety disorders. Approximately three-quarters of all agoraphobics are women. Women with agoraphobia may develop a panic attack when placed in such common situations as using public transportation (buses, airplanes, trains), being in public places like department stores, shopping malls, and crowded restaurants, or being in confined spaces such as tunnels. In all these cases, an overriding concern is the fear of being trapped in a place where escape is difficult and being overcome by a panic attack. Many women are also concerned about the reactions people around them may have if a panic attack occurs.

As the phobia becomes worse, even thinking about being in a situation to which one has a phobic reaction can engender panic. As a result, women with agoraphobia often begin to restrict their range of activities and locations. In extreme cases, they may only venture out when accompanied by a trusted friend or relative. Some agoraphobics are even afraid to be alone in their own homes unless a companion remains with them. Luckily, agoraphobia is an easily treated condition if the appropriate therapy is undertaken. A combination of medication, counseling, and stress management training will produce good results in as many as 90 percent of all people suffering from this condition.

Another common type of phobia is social phobia. This occurs when there is fear of performing in front of other people or being scrutinized by other people. The most common social phobia involves public speaking. This is a major issue for many people, including students giving speeches in class, women who must give a formal presentation at work or at social or charitable functions, and even professional actors and other performers. Other common social phobias include fear of eating in public, fear of being watched or looked at while at social gatherings, fear of signing documents in front of other people, fear of being photographed in a crowded room, or even fear of blushing in public. These phobias may begin in childhood and can persist throughout adult life (although in many women, social phobias decrease in severity with age). They often develop in children who are more shy and self-conscious.

Many people employ a variety of self help techniques to deal with social phobias, some of which are remarkably effective. For example, professional and amateur speaking groups and organizations give people the chance to speak in front of a supportive peer group; this often helps decrease anxiety related to public speaking. Classes on self-image and self-esteem utilize a variety of imaging and assertiveness techniques; these classes tend to be very popular and well-attended. Some women find that they can effectively dispel social phobias when engaged in one-on-one counseling.

A third type of phobia, called simple phobia, involves fear of a particular situation or object. Common examples of simple phobias include fear of animals like dogs or snakes, airplanes (for fear the airplane will crash), heights, or even having blood drawn for a medical test. Many simple phobias originate in childhood and persist into adult life (even though the adult may recognize that they are irrational). They may also originate in a traumatic event, such as being stuck in an elevator or experiencing a near accident during plane travel. A traumatic event may condition a person to fear repeated exposure to a similar situation (e.g., plane travel or using an elevator). Simple phobias are easiest to treat, because the fear response can usually be handled by gradual exposure to the phobia-inducing situation or object as well as the practice of a variety of stress-reducing techniques such as visualizations and affirmations. These are discussed in the self help section of this book.

Risk Factors for Anxiety Disorders

A variety of factors can predispose a woman to develop anxiety disorders. These include physiological imbalances, genetic factors (familial predisposition), family programming, major long- and short-term life stresses, and personal belief systems.

Physiological Imbalances

Research suggests that women with generalized anxiety disorder may have an imbalance of gamma amino butyric acid (GABA) in their brain. GABA is a neurotransmitter, a substance that transmits messages from one part of the brain to another. When people are given GABA or placed on drugs that increase the activity of GABA, their anxiety is diminished. While the exact mechanism triggering generalized anxiety is not known, it is possible that a GABA deficiency or extreme sensitivity on the part of the body to the available GABA levels may play a role in its etiology. Similarly, panic disorders have been identified as occurring in animals when there is a dysfunction in a specific system in the brain called the noradrenergic system. This system is very sensitive to another neurotransmitter called norepinephrine. When there is a dysfunction in the way the noradrenergic system functions, panic attacks are triggered.

Genetic Factors (Familial Predisposition)

Genetic factors seem to have some relevance as risk factors for developing anxiety disorders. For example, in studies of identical twins, the likelihood of both twins having an anxiety disorder if one is afflicted is statistically significant (greater than 30 percent). Fraternal twins, who do not have the same genetic makeup, are also at higher risk of developing an anxiety disorder if their sibling is affected, although they do not have nearly the risk of identical twins. Agoraphobia, the most common anxiety disorder, also seems to show a familial predisposition. While 5 percent of the entire population suffers from this condition, the rate of agoraphobia in people with one parent who had this diagnosis is 15 to 25 percent.

Family Programming

Certain types of family environments seem to predispose children to develop anxiety disorders, producing insecurity, fear, and dependency in susceptible children. One such setting is created by parents who are critical perfectionists, constantly demanding that a child perform at peak levels. In this family, any departure from peak performance is punished or criticized. A child in this situation may grow up with a poor sense of self-esteem, anxious and afraid to take risks for fear of failing.

Parents who themselves have phobias or are overly anxious may also raise children who suffer from anxiety. These parents tend to teach their children that the world is a fearful place, full of danger and risks. This type of family may raise a child who is timid and anxious about meeting new life challenges.

Parents who are overly controlling and suppress a child's self-assertiveness by punishment may engender anxiety in their children. In this environment, children are punished for speaking out and expressing their feelings. Such children may grow up afraid to take initiative or show their true convictions.

Not all children raised in stressful family environments develop anxiety disorders. Many children grow up in very difficult family environments without ever suffering excessive anxiety. The likelihood of developing an anxiety disorder when raised in a high-stress family is probably greater in children born with more sensitive and reactive personalities. These are children whose fight-or-flight response is easily triggered by upsetting circumstances.

Major Life Stresses

Women who have suffered from major life stresses over a long period of time, such as marriage to an abusive husband, death, chronic illness in several family members, or constant financial worries, may find their ability to handle stress with equanimity and calm hampered. Unremitting major life stresses are likely to cause wear and tear on the nervous system and, over time, cause a woman to be excessively anxious or tense.

In addition, a major stress occurring in a short period of time can also engender anxiety. This is particularly true when the stressor—such as death of a spouse or loss of a long-term job—causes significant life change or dislocation. Even positive experiences such as getting married or having a baby cause anxiety, because they throw people into entirely new situations for which they may have no preparation.

Personal Belief Systems

Many women have belief systems that reinforce the anxiety disorders and engender behavior that maintains the anxiety state. These include poor self-image and a low estimate of one's abilities. Many women with anxiety disorders are very insecure and feel ill-equipped to make the life changes necessary to confront and change anxiety-related issues.

Women with anxiety disorders often hold a negative view of the world. They see life situations and places as dangerous and threatening, whereas women without anxiety disorders may see the same circumstances as harmless and benign. These negative belief systems about the outside world, if too ingrained, may make it difficult to change.

In addition, women with anxiety disorders often reinforce their own upset through their internal dialogue. A woman who engages in constant fearful and anxious self-talk may anticipate certain situations and people as threatening and dangerous, thus reinforcing her feelings of anxiety. Because we are all constantly dialoguing with ourselves throughout much of the day, negative self-talk can be a big factor in perpetuating anxiety disorders.

In summary, anxiety disorders can take a variety of forms, including generalized anxiety disorder, panic disorder, and phobias. Many circumstances can increase the risk of developing an anxiety disorder, such as physiological imbalances, genetic factors, family upbringing, major long- and short-term life stress, and the person's own personal beliefs and negative self-talk, which can keep an anxiety disorder going once it has become an established process. Anxiety disorders can be treated through counseling, stress management techniques and breathing exercises, nutritional therapies, and regular exercise. These are discussed in depth in the self help chapters of this book.

Anxiety Due to Endocrine Imbalances

Many endocrine-related health problems have anxiety and mood swings as major symptoms. These health conditions are discussed in this section.

Premenstrual Syndrome

Anxiety and mood swings are the hallmark of premenstrual syndrome (PMS), one of the most common problems affecting women during their reproductive years (from the teens to the early fifties). In my practice, more than 90 percent of women with PMS complain of heightened anxiety and irritability that increases in intensity the week or two prior to menstruation. Many PMS patients describe severe personality changes—much like Dr. Jekyll and Mr. Hyde. They say they are irritable, witchy, and mean, that they yell at their children, pick fights with their spouses, and snap at friends and co-workers. Some spend the rest of the month repairing the emotional damage done to their relationships during this time.

Because PMS affects one-third to one-half of American women between the ages of 20 and 50 (as many as 10 to 14 million women), it is a common cause of anxiety as well as of other emotional symptoms like depression and fatigue.

In addition to the emotional symptoms, PMS has numerous physical symptoms involving almost every system in the body. More than 150 symptoms have been documented, including headaches, bloating, breast tenderness, weight gain, sugar craving, and acne. However, for many women, the emotional symptoms and fatigue are the most severe, adversely affecting their family relationships and their ability to work. In addition, it is not unusual for women to have as many as 10 or 12 of the symptoms.

There is no single cause of PMS; medical researchers now believe that various hormonal and chemical imbalances can trigger PMS symptoms. Though it is not entirely known what causes the anxiety symptoms, research suggests that several types of imbalances are likely culprits. One possible cause is an imbalance in the body's estrogen and progesterone levels. Both estrogen and progesterone increase during the second half of the menstrual cycle. Their chemical actions affect the function of almost every organ system in the body. When properly balanced, estrogen and progesterone promote healthy and balanced emotions. However, PMS mood symptoms may occur if the balance between these hormones is abnormal, because they have an opposing effect on the chemistry of the brain. Estrogen acts as a stimulant and progesterone has a sedative effect on the nervous system, so if estrogen predominates, women tend to feel anxious; and if progesterone predominates, women tend to feel depressed. Other examples of the opposing effects of estrogen and progesterone include the following: estrogen lowers blood sugar, progesterone elevates it; estrogen promotes synthesis of fats in the tissues, progesterone breaks them down. Thus, when estrogen and progesterone are appropriately balanced, women are more likely to have normal mood and behavioral patterns.

The balance between these hormones depends on two things: how much hormone the body produces, and how efficiently the body breaks it down and disposes of it. The ovaries are the primary source of estrogen and progesterone in premenopausal women (with estrogen also being synthesized by intestinal bacteria and by conversion of adrenal hormones to estrogen by the fatty tissues); the liver has the major responsibility for inactivating estrogen. The liver tries to make sure the levels of estrogen circulating through the body in a chemically active form don't become too high.

Breakdown in the liver's ability to perform this function affects the levels of estrogen in the body. Both emotional stress and your nutritional habits play significant roles in how efficiently this system will run. For example, excessive intake of fats, alcohol, and sugar stresses the liver, which must process these foods as well as the hormone. With vitamin B deficiency, which can be caused by poor nutrition or by emotional stress, the liver lacks the raw material to carry out its metabolic tasks. In either case, the liver cannot break down the hormones efficiently, so higher levels of hormones continue to circulate in the blood without proper disposal, tipping the balance toward excessive anxiety-producing estrogen.

Other research studies link the emotional symptoms of PMS to chemical imbalances in the central nervous system. Some researchers suggest that the symptoms of anxiety and mood swings are due to a heightened sensitivity in some women to fluctuations in the body's level of beta endorphins. These substances are the body's natural opiates, producing a sense of well-being and even elation when present in large amounts. (Beta endorphins are responsible for the "runner's high" that many people experience after prolonged aerobic exercise, because exercise increases beta endorphin production.) Beta endorphin levels increase soon after ovulation at mid-cycle and may decline with the approach of menstruation. A fall in beta endorphin levels in women who are very sensitive to the effects of these chemicals or who produce large amounts of beta endorphin could, like opiate withdrawal, cause symptoms such as anxiety and irritability.

Another possible cause of PMS anxiety symptoms may be the lack of sufficient serotonin in the brain. Serotonin is a neurotransmitter that regulates rapid eye movement (REM) sleep and appetite. Inadequate levels of serotonin could explain the poor sleep quality with the resultant fatigue, anxiety, and irritability from which some women with PMS suffer. It could also explain, at least in part, why some women with PMS feel that they have such a difficult time controlling their eating habits and managing their food cravings during the premenstrual time. Serotonin is produced in the body from an amino acid called tryptophan. Tryptophan is an essential amino acid that must be replaced daily through adequate dietary intake since our body cannot manufacture it from other sources. Good sources of tryptophan include almonds, pumpkin seeds, and sesame seeds.

Many factors increase the risk of PMS in susceptible women. PMS occurs most frequently in women over 30; the most severe symptoms occur in women in their thirties and forties. Women are at high risk when they are under significant emotional stress or if they have poor nutritional habits and don't exercise. Women who are unable to tolerate birth control pills seem to be more likely to suffer PMS, as are women who have had a pregnancy complicated by toxemia. Also, the more children a woman has, the more severe her PMS symptoms.

PMS rarely goes away spontaneously without treatment. My experience is that it gets worse with age. Some of my most uncomfortable patients are women in their middle to late forties who are also approaching menopause. These women often feel they have the worst of both life phases as they pass from their reproductive years into menopause. Often, PMS symptoms coexist with bleeding irregularities and hot flashes. Once the PMS is treated, the accompanying fatigue and mood symptoms clear up. Therapies for PMS are discussed in the self help section of this book.

As mentioned earlier, no single hormonal or chemical imbalance has been linked to PMS. Instead, nearly two dozen hormonal, chemical, and nutritional imbalances may contribute to causing the symptoms. Even more confusing for patients and physicians alike is that the underlying causes may differ from one woman to another. As a result, no single wonder drug cures PMS, although many drugs have been tested, including hormones, tranquilizers, antidepressants, and diuretics. Luckily, the anxiety and mood swing symptoms of PMS as well as the physical symptoms respond very well to healthful lifestyle changes. In my practice, I have found PMS to be a very treatable problem. Achieving results does, however, require that women participate actively in their own program, adopt good nutritional habits, and deal with stress more effectively.

Menopause

Menopause, the end of all menstrual bleeding, occurs for most women between the ages of 48 and 52. However, some women cease menstruating as young as their late thirties or early forties, while others continue to menstruate into their mid-fifties. Anxiety, mood swings, and fatigue often accompany this process as women go through the hormonal changes that lead to the cessation of menstruation.

For most women, the transition to menopause occurs gradually, triggered by a slowdown in the function of their ovaries. The process begins four to six years before the last menstrual period and continues for several years after. During this period of transition, estrogen production from the ovaries decreases, eventually dropping to such low levels that menstruation becomes irregular and finally ceases entirely. For some women this transition to a new, lower level of hormonal equilibrium is easy and uneventful. For many women, however, the transition is difficult, fraught with many uncomfortable symptoms, such as irregular bleeding, hot flashes, anxiety, mood swings, and fatigue. As many as 80 percent of women going through menopause experience some of these symptoms.

In my medical practice, I have seen many women who experienced marked emotional symptoms while going through menopause. In fact, many of my patients have described symptoms similar to those of PMS. The psychological symptoms of menopause include insomnia (often associated with hot flashes), irritability, anxiety, depression, and fatigue. As mentioned in the section on PMS, both estrogen and progesterone have been studied for their effects on mood: If estrogen predominates, women tend to feel anxious; if progesterone predominates, women may feel depressed and tired. As women go through menopause, there is first an imbalance in these hormones and finally a deficiency in both as their ovarian production drops to very low levels or ceases entirely. The severity of the symptoms probably depends on the individual woman's biochemistry and on psychosocial factors. Women have worse symptoms if they are under severe emotional stress or have aggravating dietary habits, such as excessive caffeine, sugar, or alcohol intake.

The emotional symptoms of menopause can also be aggravated by lifestyle issues. For some women, the social and cultural factors occurring before, during, and after menopause may be quite stressful. Menopause can be a time when children leave home and move away, major career changes are made, and marriage ends in divorce or starts anew. Of course, these major life changes can occur at other times besides the "mid-life crisis," but the combination of hormonal and biochemical changes plus lifestyle changes can be quite difficult to handle.

There are many effective treatments to reduce the emotional and physical symptoms of menopause. These include hormonal replacement therapy and, in more severe cases, the use of mood-altering drugs. Vitamin, herbal, and mineral supplements help support menopausal women's reproductive and glandular systems. Stress-management techniques and regular exercise may also help restore energy and vitality and stabilize mood. These are discussed in the self help section of this book.

Hyperthyroidism

When the thyroid gland excretes an excessive amount of thyroid hormone, hyperthyroidism occurs. This is a potentially serious and dangerous problem if not diagnosed right away. Symptoms of hyperthyroidism can mimic those of anxiety attacks, and include generalized anxiety, insomnia, easy fatigability, rapid heartbeat, sweating, heat intolerance, and loose bowel movements. In fact, the correct diagnosis may often be missed initially, especially with women who are in menopause, if the symptoms are thought to be due simply to stress or the change of life.

Hyperthyroidism does, however, present with other symptoms that should tip off both the woman and her physician that there is a physiological imbalance present. These symptoms include weight loss despite a ravenous appetite, quick movements, trembling of the hands, and difficulty focusing the eyes. On a medical examination, many signs of hyperthyroidism may also be present. The skin of a woman with this problem is usually warm and moist. A goiter (enlargement of the thyroid) may be felt by the physician. The skin and hair are usually thin and silky in texture. The eyes usually tend to stare, and in more advanced cases, even bulge from the eye sockets. In advanced cases, there is also muscle wasting and bone loss (osteoporosis) as well as heart abnormalities. As you can see, hyperthyroidism causes severe and potentially dangerous changes in the body and should be considered when trying to diagnose the cause of anxiety episodes.

A diagnosis of hyperthyroidism can be made early by blood tests that show excessive secretion of thyroid hormones, as well as other changes in the blood. If heart and bone abnormalities are present also, they may show on an electrocardiograph and on x-rays. Once diagnosed, hyperthyroidism should be treated immediately to reduce the hormonal output. Treatments include the use of drugs that suppress and even inactivate the thyroid gland, as well as surgical removal of the thyroid. This is discussed in detail in Chapter 11 of this book.

Women with thyroid dysfunction often have exhaustion in other endocrine glands. The adrenal glands are particularly affected by poor thyroid function, as well as any other physical and emotional stress. The adrenals are two almond-sized glands that secrete several dozen hormones. One of these is cortisol, an important hormone that helps regulate our response to stress. Stress can be a response to strong emotional feelings, such as anxiety or depression, or to physical triggers, such as an allergic reaction, infectious disease, burns, surgery, or an accident. Whatever the source of stress, cortisol lessens its injurious effects on the body, reducing pain, swelling, and fever.

When stress has been recurrent and of long duration, the adrenal glands can become exhausted, mustering less and less ability to buffer the negative effects of physical and emotional stress. As a result of adrenal exhaustion, the individual may experience an increase in fatigue and tiredness. Much rest, stress management, and nutritional support are required to restore the adrenals and rebuild the physiological "cushion" to deal with stress. There are many helpful techniques listed in the self help section of this book to help restore the glandular system.

Hypoglycemia

This condition occurs when the blood sugar levels in the body fall too low. With this condition, people experience many symptoms similar to those of anxiety attacks, including anxiety, irritability, trembling, disorientation, light-headedness, spaciness, and even palpitations. The dietary trigger for hypoglycemia episodes is excessive intake of simple sugars such as white sugar, honey, fruit juice, white flour products, and sugar-laden desserts such as cookies, doughnuts, and candies.

Glucose, or sugar, is critical for survival because it is the major fuel our bodies run on (the brain alone uses up to 20 percent of the glucose available in the body to fuel its normal level of functioning). However, simple sugars require little processing in the digestive tract and are absorbed rapidly into the blood circulation, overloading the body with fuel. To move this abundance of sugar into the cells where it can be processed and utilized for the cells' energy needs, the hormone insulin is released from the pancreas. Without adequate insulin, sugar cannot be moved into the cells. Unfortunately, when too much sugar is dumped into the blood circulation, usually the reverse situation occurs and too much insulin is secreted. This can actually drop the blood sugar too low (below 50-60 milligrams per milliliter) to levels where the typical anxiety-like symptoms of hypoglycemia occur. Interestingly, drops in the blood sugar level can also occur simply in response to heightened levels of stress, because the body utilizes extra glucose or fuel during this time.

When the blood sugar level falls too low, the brain is rapidly deprived of energy. A correction must occur in order to bring the glucose levels back to normal, so the adrenal glands release the hormones cortisol and adrenaline which cause the liver to release stored sugar. Though the stored sugar from the liver does restore the blood sugar balance, the rise in adrenal hormonal output also increases emotional arousal and anxiety. Thus, the hypoglycemia cycle can perpetuate the physical and psychological symptoms of anxiety. Women who continue to eat a diet high in simple sugar often feel as though they are on an emotional roller coaster, tossed from highs to lows of anxiety and irritability on the one hand and fatigue and depression on the other, as their blood sugar levels fluctuate.

Most women can easily solve this problem by switching to a diet high in complex carbohydrate foods. These include whole grains, starches, whole fruits, and vegetables. When eaten by themselves or when combined with high-quality proteins such as nuts, seeds, and fish, the complex carbohydrates are broken down to glucose and slowly absorbed into the blood circulation, thus not triggering excessive insulin output. As a result, both the blood sugar level and the emotions stay healthy and balanced. In addition, consuming proper vitamins and minerals supports glucose metabolism and pancreatic function, thereby preventing symptoms in women prone to hypoglycemia-related anxiety attacks. Both the optimal diet and nutritional supplements for hypoglycemia are discussed in the self help chapters of this book.

Anxiety Due to Immune System Imbalances

Immune system disorders can cause a variety of psychological as well as physical symptoms. These imbalances are discussed in detail in this section.

Allergies, Including Food Allergies

Many women are unaware that allergic reactions can cause mood changes such as anxiety. Allergies occur when the body's immune system overreacts to harmless substances. Normally, the immune system is on the alert for invaders such as viruses, bacteria, and other organisms that cause disease. The immune system's job is to identify these invaders and to produce antibodies which destroy them before they cause illness. In allergic people, this system begins to react to other substances—typically pollens, molds, or foods. Common food allergens include wheat, milk (and milk products), alcohol, chocolate, eggs, yeast, peanuts, citrus fruits, tomatoes, corn, and shellfish.

Sometimes allergic reactions are easily diagnosed, because the symptoms occur immediately after the encounter with the allergen.

Immediate allergic symptoms include wheezing, itching and tearing of the eyes, nasal congestion, and hives. Some allergic reactions are delayed; they may occur hours or days after exposure to the allergen. Delayed symptoms include anxiety, depression, fatigue, dizziness, spaciness, headaches, joint and muscle aches and pains, and eczema. Food allergies can also affect digestive function, causing inflammation of the intestinal lining and pain in the abdominal area. Damage to the intestinal lining causes it to become more porous and permeable. When large particles of poorly digested food, to which the person is allergic, are absorbed into the body, the body's defense system is activated, precipitating damage to many organs and tissues by autoantibodies. (These are the immune complexes that attack your own tissues as if they were foreign substances.) The person affected may be unaware that an allergy is causing her emotional and physical symptoms. This often occurs with food allergies, as well as with a variety of chemical triggers.

Food allergies commonly trigger anxiety episodes in susceptible women. Often, you crave the foods to which you are allergic. Thus, food addiction may actually be a sign of food allergy. Women commonly crave foods such as chocolate, chips, pasta, bread, and milk products. Often they find that once they start eating these foods, they have a difficult time stopping. A woman who has the desire to have one chocolate can end up eating a whole box. The decision to eat one cookie can turn into a binge of ten or fifteen at one session, or a small dish of ice cream becomes a pint. Though binging tendencies can be seen throughout the month in women with food allergies, they tend to be worse during the premenstrual period (which may commence as early as two weeks prior to the onset of menstruation). Alterations in mood as well as physical symptoms typical of anxiety, such as increased heart rate and respiration, often coexist with the food craving symptom.

Some holistic physicians test for food allergies by doing sublingual provocative tests. In this test, a food extract is placed under the tongue to see whether it elicits a reaction. Neutralizing antidotes are then administered to the patient to reduce or eliminate symptoms. This test is not used by traditional allergists, who consider it to be ineffective. Another way to test for food sensitivities is simply to eliminate suspected food allergens. First, the patient fasts, taking only distilled water for several days. Then she reintroduces foods one at a time. If the patient is allergic to a specific food, a reaction will occur after she adds that food to her diet. Another method is to maintain a low-stress diet and to eliminate only the particular food to which you suspect you may be allergic, again reintroducing these foods sequentially to see how your body reacts. You may actually feel worse initially after eliminating high-stress foods, due to the withdrawal symptoms that occur after stopping anything to which you are addicted. (This can also happen when stopping drugs and cigarettes.) During the period when you are determining your food allergies, keep a diary in which you record your emotional and physical symptoms, both on and off the offending foods. This will help you evaluate the severity of your reactions. Finally, there is a blood test now available called the RAST test; while quite expensive, it gives the physician a complete profile of allergens, including foods, pollens, flowers, grasses, and so forth.

Treatment for food and other allergies usually includes avoiding the offending substance, if possible, or using over-the-counter and prescription medication and desensitization shots. Managing stress and following a low-stress elimination diet may also help treat and prevent allergies. It is important to rotate foods and choose from a wide variety of high-nutrient food. Certain nutritional supplements also help to support and strengthen the immune system. These topics are discussed in the self help section of this book.

Anxiety Due to Cardiovascular System Disorders

While cardiovascular problems primarily cause physical symptoms, mitral valve prolapse can cause psychological symptoms as well.

Mitral Valve Prolapse

Mitral valve prolapse is a heart condition that can cause anxiety-like episodes of palpitations, chest pain, shortness of breath, and fatigue. It does appear to be present more frequently in people with anxiety and panic episodes than in the general population. It is caused by a mild defect in the mitral valve, which is located between the upper and lower chamber on the left side of the heart. Normally, blood flows unimpeded between the two chambers. However, with mitral valve prolapse, the valve doesn't close completely. As a result, the heart is put under stress and can beat either too fast or erratically.

In more severe cases, the heartbeat can be slowed through the use of beta blockers, drugs that decrease heart rate and heart contractility by decreasing oxygen consumption. (This is discussed in detail in Chapter 11 of this book.) In addition, undue stress and stimulants such as caffeine-containing beverages like coffee, tea, and cola drinks should be eliminated in order to avoid triggering episodes of rapid heartbeat. Deficiencies of calcium, magnesium, and potassium should be avoided since these essential minerals help to regulate and reduce cardiac irritability. To ensure adequate daily intake, it is important to maintain a diet with sufficient amounts of these nutrients or to use supplements.

Common Causes of Anxiety

Types of anxiety disorders
Generalized anxiety disorder
Panic disorder
Phobias

Physical conditions associated with anxiety

Premenstrual syndrome	Hypoglycemia
Menopause	Food allergies
Hyperthyroidism	Mitral valve prolapse

Evaluating
Your Symptoms

2

The Anxiety & Stress Workbook

During the many years that I have worked with anxiety relief self help programs, I have found that a woman's own evaluation of her symptoms is as important as the actual treatments. Often, a personal evaluation of the problems by the woman herself helps to clarify the types of symptoms as well as their severity in her own mind. Self-evaluation also helps a woman to become aware of possible risk factors based on her lifestyle habits, as well as the existence of health problems that can trigger anxiety symptoms and may have gone undiagnosed. The woman can also share this information with her health-care provider, thereby providing more complete data when a medical exam is performed. I have personally found it very helpful when my patients share the following charts with me.

This workbook section can help you evaluate many of the factors that contribute to anxiety and stress. First, begin to fill out the monthly calendar of anxiety and stress symptoms, starting today. If you recall your symptoms for the past month, chart these symptoms as well. The calendar will allow you to see which types of symptoms you have, as well as evaluate their severity. This will make it easier for you to pick the specific treatments for symptom relief. Then, as you follow the program, you can keep using the monthly calendars (a year's worth have been included) to check your progress.

Monthly Calendar of Anxiety Symptoms

Grade your symptoms as you experience them each month: ○ None ✓ Mild ◗ Moderate ▲ Severe

Symptom

Symptom	1	2	3	4	5	6	7	8	9	10
Excessive tension or nervousness										
Feelings of being on edge										
Easily startled, jumpy										
Difficulty falling or staying asleep										
Easily angered, irritable										
Restlessness, easily excited										
Dizziness, shakiness, tremulousness										
Difficulty concentrating or focusing										
Blue moods alternating with anxiety										
Excessive tiredness or fatigue										
Fear of certain locations, situations										
Fear of other people										
Frequent nightmares										
Muscle tightness or tension										
Fast or irregular heartbeat										
Chest pain										
Shortness of breath										
Excessive sweating										
Dry mouth										
Intestinal cramps, nausea, diarrhea										
Frequent urination										
Hot flashes or feeling of chilliness										
Cold hands and feet										
Tightness in throat or lump in throat										

DAY OF MONTH

Month 1 _____

11	12	13	14	15	16	17	18	19	20	21	22	23	24	25	26	27	28	29	30	31

Monthly Calendar of Anxiety Symptoms

Grade your symptoms as you experience them each
month: ○ None ✓ Mild ◗ Moderate ▲ Severe

Symptom

Symptom	1	2	3	4	5	6	7	8	9	10
Excessive tension or nervousness										
Feelings of being on edge										
Easily startled, jumpy										
Difficulty falling or staying asleep										
Easily angered, irritable										
Restlessness, easily excited										
Dizziness, shakiness, tremulousness										
Difficulty concentrating or focusing										
Blue moods alternating with anxiety										
Excessive tiredness or fatigue										
Fear of certain locations, situations										
Fear of other people										
Frequent nightmares										
Muscle tightness or tension										
Fast or irregular heartbeat										
Chest pain										
Shortness of breath										
Excessive sweating										
Dry mouth										
Intestinal cramps, nausea, diarrhea										
Frequent urination										
Hot flashes or feeling of chilliness										
Cold hands and feet										
Tightness in throat or lump in throat										

Month 2 _____

11	12	13	14	15	16	17	18	19	20	21	22	23	24	25	26	27	28	29	30	31

Monthly Calendar of Anxiety Symptoms

Grade your symptoms as you experience them each
month: ◯ None ✓ Mild ◗ Moderate ▲ Severe

Symptom

Symptom	DAY OF MONTH									
	1	2	3	4	5	6	7	8	9	10
Excessive tension or nervousness										
Feelings of being on edge										
Easily startled, jumpy										
Difficulty falling or staying asleep										
Easily angered, irritable										
Restlessness, easily excited										
Dizziness, shakiness, tremulousness										
Difficulty concentrating or focusing										
Blue moods alternating with anxiety										
Excessive tiredness or fatigue										
Fear of certain locations, situations										
Fear of other people										
Frequent nightmares										
Muscle tightness or tension										
Fast or irregular heartbeat										
Chest pain										
Shortness of breath										
Excessive sweating										
Dry mouth										
Intestinal cramps, nausea, diarrhea										
Frequent urination										
Hot flashes or feeling of chilliness										
Cold hands and feet										
Tightness in throat or lump in throat										

DAY OF MONTH   **Month 3** _____

11	12	13	14	15	16	17	18	19	20	21	22	23	24	25	26	27	28	29	30	31

Monthly Calendar of Anxiety Symptoms

Grade your symptoms as you experience them each month: ○ None ✓ Mild ◗ Moderate ▲ Severe

Symptom

Symptom	1	2	3	4	5	6	7	8	9	10
Excessive tension or nervousness										
Feelings of being on edge										
Easily startled, jumpy										
Difficulty falling or staying asleep										
Easily angered, irritable										
Restlessness, easily excited										
Dizziness, shakiness, tremulousness										
Difficulty concentrating or focusing										
Blue moods alternating with anxiety										
Excessive tiredness or fatigue										
Fear of certain locations, situations										
Fear of other people										
Frequent nightmares										
Muscle tightness or tension										
Fast or irregular heartbeat										
Chest pain										
Shortness of breath										
Excessive sweating										
Dry mouth										
Intestinal cramps, nausea, diarrhea										
Frequent urination										
Hot flashes or feeling of chilliness										
Cold hands and feet										
Tightness in throat or lump in throat										

Month 4 _____

11	12	13	14	15	16	17	18	19	20	21	22	23	24	25	26	27	28	29	30	31

Monthly Calendar of Anxiety Symptoms

Grade your symptoms as you experience them each month: ○ None ✓ Mild ◗ Moderate ▲ Severe

Symptom

Symptom	DAY OF MONTH									
	1	2	3	4	5	6	7	8	9	10
Excessive tension or nervousness										
Feelings of being on edge										
Easily startled, jumpy										
Difficulty falling or staying asleep										
Easily angered, irritable										
Restlessness, easily excited										
Dizziness, shakiness, tremulousness										
Difficulty concentrating or focusing										
Blue moods alternating with anxiety										
Excessive tiredness or fatigue										
Fear of certain locations, situations										
Fear of other people										
Frequent nightmares										
Muscle tightness or tension										
Fast or irregular heartbeat										
Chest pain										
Shortness of breath										
Excessive sweating										
Dry mouth										
Intestinal cramps, nausea, diarrhea										
Frequent urination										
Hot flashes or feeling of chilliness										
Cold hands and feet										
Tightness in throat or lump in throat										

Month 5 _____

11	12	13	14	15	16	17	18	19	20	21	22	23	24	25	26	27	28	29	30	31

Monthly Calendar of Anxiety Symptoms

Grade your symptoms as you experience them each month: ○ None ✓ Mild ◗ Moderate ▲ Severe

Symptom

Excessive tension or nervousness

Feelings of being on edge

Easily startled, jumpy

Difficulty falling or staying asleep

Easily angered, irritable

Restlessness, easily excited

Dizziness, shakiness, tremulousness

Difficulty concentrating or focusing

Blue moods alternating with anxiety

Excessive tiredness or fatigue

Fear of certain locations, situations

Fear of other people

Frequent nightmares

Muscle tightness or tension

Fast or irregular heartbeat

Chest pain

Shortness of breath

Excessive sweating

Dry mouth

Intestinal cramps, nausea, diarrhea

Frequent urination

Hot flashes or feeling of chilliness

Cold hands and feet

Tightness in throat or lump in throat

DAY OF MONTH

1	2	3	4	5	6	7	8	9	10

Month 6 _____

11	12	13	14	15	16	17	18	19	20	21	22	23	24	25	26	27	28	29	30	31

Monthly Calendar of Anxiety Symptoms

Grade your symptoms as you experience them each
month: ○ None ✓ Mild ◗ Moderate ▲ Severe

Symptom

Symptom	1	2	3	4	5	6	7	8	9	10
Excessive tension or nervousness										
Feelings of being on edge										
Easily startled, jumpy										
Difficulty falling or staying asleep										
Easily angered, irritable										
Restlessness, easily excited										
Dizziness, shakiness, tremulousness										
Difficulty concentrating or focusing										
Blue moods alternating with anxiety										
Excessive tiredness or fatigue										
Fear of certain locations, situations										
Fear of other people										
Frequent nightmares										
Muscle tightness or tension										
Fast or irregular heartbeat										
Chest pain										
Shortness of breath										
Excessive sweating										
Dry mouth										
Intestinal cramps, nausea, diarrhea										
Frequent urination										
Hot flashes or feeling of chilliness										
Cold hands and feet										
Tightness in throat or lump in throat										

Month 7 _____

11	12	13	14	15	16	17	18	19	20	21	22	23	24	25	26	27	28	29	30	31

Monthly Calendar of Anxiety Symptoms

Grade your symptoms as you experience them each month: ○ None ✓ Mild ◗ Moderate ▲ Severe

Symptom

DAY OF MONTH									
1	2	3	4	5	6	7	8	9	10

Excessive tension or nervousness

Feelings of being on edge

Easily startled, jumpy

Difficulty falling or staying asleep

Easily angered, irritable

Restlessness, easily excited

Dizziness, shakiness, tremulousness

Difficulty concentrating or focusing

Blue moods alternating with anxiety

Excessive tiredness or fatigue

Fear of certain locations, situations

Fear of other people

Frequent nightmares

Muscle tightness or tension

Fast or irregular heartbeat

Chest pain

Shortness of breath

Excessive sweating

Dry mouth

Intestinal cramps, nausea, diarrhea

Frequent urination

Hot flashes or feeling of chilliness

Cold hands and feet

Tightness in throat or lump in throat

Month 8 _____

11	12	13	14	15	16	17	18	19	20	21	22	23	24	25	26	27	28	29	30	31

Monthly Calendar of Anxiety Symptoms

Grade your symptoms as you experience them each month: ○ None ✓ Mild ◗ Moderate ▲ Severe

Symptom

Symptom	1	2	3	4	5	6	7	8	9	10
Excessive tension or nervousness										
Feelings of being on edge										
Easily startled, jumpy										
Difficulty falling or staying asleep										
Easily angered, irritable										
Restlessness, easily excited										
Dizziness, shakiness, tremulousness										
Difficulty concentrating or focusing										
Blue moods alternating with anxiety										
Excessive tiredness or fatigue										
Fear of certain locations, situations										
Fear of other people										
Frequent nightmares										
Muscle tightness or tension										
Fast or irregular heartbeat										
Chest pain										
Shortness of breath										
Excessive sweating										
Dry mouth										
Intestinal cramps, nausea, diarrhea										
Frequent urination										
Hot flashes or feeling of chilliness										
Cold hands and feet										
Tightness in throat or lump in throat										

11	12	13	14	15	16	17	18	19	20	21	22	23	24	25	26	27	28	29	30	31

Monthly Calendar of Anxiety Symptoms

Grade your symptoms as you experience them each
month: ○ None ✓ Mild ◗ Moderate ▲ Severe

Symptom

	1	2	3	4	5	6	7	8	9	10
DAY OF MONTH										
Excessive tension or nervousness										
Feelings of being on edge										
Easily startled, jumpy										
Difficulty falling or staying asleep										
Easily angered, irritable										
Restlessness, easily excited										
Dizziness, shakiness, tremulousness										
Difficulty concentrating or focusing										
Blue moods alternating with anxiety										
Excessive tiredness or fatigue										
Fear of certain locations, situations										
Fear of other people										
Frequent nightmares										
Muscle tightness or tension										
Fast or irregular heartbeat										
Chest pain										
Shortness of breath										
Excessive sweating										
Dry mouth										
Intestinal cramps, nausea, diarrhea										
Frequent urination										
Hot flashes or feeling of chilliness										
Cold hands and feet										
Tightness in throat or lump in throat										

Month 10 _____

11	12	13	14	15	16	17	18	19	20	21	22	23	24	25	26	27	28	29	30	31

Monthly Calendar of Anxiety Symptoms

Grade your symptoms as you experience them each month: ○ None ✓ Mild ◗ Moderate ▲ Severe

Symptom

Symptom	1	2	3	4	5	6	7	8	9	10
Excessive tension or nervousness										
Feelings of being on edge										
Easily startled, jumpy										
Difficulty falling or staying asleep										
Easily angered, irritable										
Restlessness, easily excited										
Dizziness, shakiness, tremulousness										
Difficulty concentrating or focusing										
Blue moods alternating with anxiety										
Excessive tiredness or fatigue										
Fear of certain locations, situations										
Fear of other people										
Frequent nightmares										
Muscle tightness or tension										
Fast or irregular heartbeat										
Chest pain										
Shortness of breath										
Excessive sweating										
Dry mouth										
Intestinal cramps, nausea, diarrhea										
Frequent urination										
Hot flashes or feeling of chilliness										
Cold hands and feet										
Tightness in throat or lump in throat										

Month 11 _____

11	12	13	14	15	16	17	18	19	20	21	22	23	24	25	26	27	28	29	30	31

Monthly Calendar of Anxiety Symptoms

Grade your symptoms as you experience them each month: ○ None ✓ Mild ◗ Moderate ▲ Severe

Symptom

	1	2	3	4	5	6	7	8	9	10
Excessive tension or nervousness										
Feelings of being on edge										
Easily startled, jumpy										
Difficulty falling or staying asleep										
Easily angered, irritable										
Restlessness, easily excited										
Dizziness, shakiness, tremulousness										
Difficulty concentrating or focusing										
Blue moods alternating with anxiety										
Excessive tiredness or fatigue										
Fear of certain locations, situations										
Fear of other people										
Frequent nightmares										
Muscle tightness or tension										
Fast or irregular heartbeat										
Chest pain										
Shortness of breath										
Excessive sweating										
Dry mouth										
Intestinal cramps, nausea, diarrhea										
Frequent urination										
Hot flashes or feeling of chilliness										
Cold hands and feet										
Tightness in throat or lump in throat										

Month 12 _____

11	12	13	14	15	16	17	18	19	20	21	22	23	24	25	26	27	28	29	30	31

After you've filled out the calendar, turn to the risk factor and lifestyle evaluations that follow. They will help you assess specific areas of your life to see which of your habit patterns may be contributing to your health problems. Lifestyle habits impact the symptoms of anxiety and stress significantly. By filling out the workbook sheets, you can easily recognize your weak areas. When you've completed the evaluations, you will be ready to go on to the self help chapters and begin your treatment program.

Risk Factors for Anxiety

You are at higher risk for developing symptoms of anxiety and stress if you have any of the risk factors listed below. Be sure to follow the nutritional, exercise, and stress management guidelines in the self help section of this book if you have any of the related risk factors for anxiety listed here. Place a check beside each risk factor that applies to you.

Risk Factors

Relatives with a history of anxiety disorders, phobias,   ____
    or agoraphobia

History of overly critical parents, lack of emotional nurturing   ____

History of parents who suppressed and punished and   ____
    communication and verbalization of feelings

History of fearful and overly cautious parents   ____

History of fearing separation from parents in childhood   ____
    (going to school, play activities, or even falling
    asleep without parents)

Significant life stress such as death, illness, or divorce   ____
    preceding onset of excessive anxiety

PMS   ____

Menopause   ____

Hyperthyroidism (excessive thyroid function)   ____

Hypoglycemia   ____

Food allergies or allergy to food additives (such as aspartame) ____

Food addictions ____

Mitral valve prolapse ____

Use of estrogen-containing medication ____

Withdrawal from alcohol, tranquilizers, or sedatives ____

Use of recreational drugs (such as cocaine, amphetamines) ____
   that increase anxiety levels

Excessive use of coffee, black tea, colas, chocolates, or other ____
   caffeine-containing foods

Excessive use of sugar ____

Calcium, magnesium, or potassium deficiency ____

Lack of B vitamins ____

Eating Habits Evaluation

Check off the number of times you eat the following foods.
Foods That Increase Symptoms

Foods	Never	Once a Month	Once a Week	Twice a Week +
Cow's milk				
Cow's cheese				
Butter				
Yogurt				
Eggs				
Chocolate				
Sugar				
Alcohol				
Wheat bread				
Wheat noodles				
Wheat-based flour				
Pastries				
Added salt				
Bouillon				

Foods	Never	Once a Month	Once a Week	Twice a Week +
Commercial salad dressing				
Catsup				
Coffee				
Black tea				
Soft drinks				
Hot dogs				
Ham				
Bacon				
Beef				
Lamb				
Pork				

Foods That Decrease Symptoms

Foods	Never	Once a Month	Once a Week	Twice a Week +
Avocados				
Beans				
Beets				
Broccoli				
Brussels sprouts				
Cabbage				
Carrots				
Celery				
Collard greens				
Cucumbers				
Eggplant				
Garlic				
Horseradish				
Kale				
Lettuce				
Mustard greens				
Okra				
Onions				

Foods	Never	Once a Month	Once a Week	Twice a Week +
Parsnips				
Peas				
Potatoes				
Radishes				
Rutabagas				
Spinach				
Squash				
Sweet potatoes				
Tomatoes				
Turnips				
Turnip greens				
Yams				
Brown rice				
Millet				
Barley				
Oatmeal				
Buckwheat				
Rye				
Corn				
Raw flax seeds				
Raw pumpkin seeds				
Raw sesame seeds				
Raw sunflower seeds				
Raw almonds				
Raw filberts				
Raw pecans				
Raw walnuts				
Apples				
Bananas				
Berries				
Pears				
Seasonal fruits				

Foods	Never	Once a Month	Once a Week	Twice a Week +
Corn oil				
Flax oil				
Olive oil				
Sesame oil				
Safflower oil				
Poultry				
Fish				

Key to Eating Habits

All the foods in the shaded area are unhealthy foods that can increase the symptoms of anxiety and stress. In addition, many of these foods tend to worsen your health in general and should be avoided. If you eat many of these foods, or if you eat any of these foods frequently, your nutritional habits may be contributing significantly to your symptoms. For further guidance on food selection, refer to Chapters 3 and 4.

The foods listed in the unshaded area, from avocados to fish, are high-nutrient, low-stress foods that may help relieve or prevent anxiety and stress symptoms. Include these foods frequently in your diet. If you are already eating many of these and few of the high-stress foods, chances are your nutritional habits are good, and food selection may not be a significant factor in worsening your symptoms. You may want to look carefully at the stress-management and exercise chapters. The activities contained in these chapters may be very helpful in relieving your symptoms.

Exercises Habits

Check the frequency with which you do any of the following:

Activity	Never	Once a Month	1 or 2x a Week	3x a Week +
Jogging				
Walking				
Bicycling				
Skiing				
Swimming				
Aerobic dancing				
Jumping rope				
Ice skating				
Roller skating				
Handball				
Racquetball				
Tennis				
Soccer				
Basketball				
Baseball				
Table tennis				
Golf				
Croquet				
Bowling				
Yoga				
Stretching				
Weight lifting				
Gardening				

Key to Exercise Habits

Exercise helps to relieve symptoms of anxiety and stress. It also helps to reduce the symptoms of muscular tension that often accompany the emotional distress. If your total number of exercise periods per week is less than three, you probably need to increase your level of physical activity. See Chapter 8 for recommendations on the type of exercise that would be best suited for you and help reduce your anxiety symptoms.

Some women with anxiety tend to over exercise. They work out with such intensity that they are actually triggering panic symptoms. If you suspect that this is what is happening to you, you may want to modify your current regimen. You will find many options available in Chapters 8, 9, and 10, on physical exercise, yoga, and acupressure.

Symptoms of Lack of Physical Fitness and Stamina

Check those symptoms that pertain to you:

	Yes	No
Fatigue, tiredness, lethargy	___	___
Tiredness or exhaustion when walking less than a mile	___	___
Shortness of breath when walking less than a mile	___	___
Tiredness or exhaustion when walking up a flight of stairs	___	___
Shortness of breath when walking up a flight of stairs	___	___
Excessive weight or obesity	___	___
Poor muscle tone	___	___
Excessive muscle tension and/or cramping when engaging in physical activity	___	___
Eyestrain	___	___
Chronic neck pain and muscle tension	___	___
Chronic shoulder and upper-middle-back tension	___	___
Grinding of teeth (bruxism)	___	___
Chronic low back pain	___	___
Chronic abdominal tension	___	___
Chronic arm tension	___	___

Key to Lack of Physical Fitness and Stamina

If you find that symptoms listed in this evaluation pertain to you, you should start a physical fitness program slowly and carefully. Your level of physical activity should be increased gradually until your body is more conditioned to the point where exercise is not as difficult to do. You may want to notify your physician regarding these symptoms. Your physician may then help guide you in designing the best exercise regimen for your needs. In addition, some of these symptoms may indicate an underlying health problem that should be evaluated.

Key to Daily Exercise Diary

This diary should help you determine if your current exercise program is right for helping reduce your anxiety and stress symptoms as well as promote optimal physical conditioning. A good exercise program should leave you feeling energized and relaxed at the same time. You should also do activities you enjoy so that you look forward to your exercise session.

In monitoring your physical responses to vigorous aerobic exercise, make sure that the session increases your pulse rate to the optimal range for your age, as follows:

Age	Pulse rate (also indicates heart rate)
20–29	145–164
30–39	138–156
40–49	130–148
50–59	122–140
60+	116–132

If, when filling out the diary, you find that your exercise program is not satisfactory, then switch to other physical activities. Read the chapters on physical exercise, yoga, and acupressure massage for other options.

Daily Exercise Diary   **Month** _____

	Date	Time	Exercise type	Session length	Pulse rate
1	____	____	_____	_____	_____
2	____	____	_____	_____	_____
3	____	____	_____	_____	_____
4	____	____	_____	_____	_____
5	____	____	_____	_____	_____
6	____	____	_____	_____	_____
7	____	____	_____	_____	_____
8	____	____	_____	_____	_____
9	____	____	_____	_____	_____
10	____	____	_____	_____	_____
11	____	____	_____	_____	_____
12	____	____	_____	_____	_____
13	____	____	_____	_____	_____
14	____	____	_____	_____	_____
15	____	____	_____	_____	_____
16	____	____	_____	_____	_____
17	____	____	_____	_____	_____
18	____	____	_____	_____	_____
19	____	____	_____	_____	_____
20	____	____	_____	_____	_____
21	____	____	_____	_____	_____
22	____	____	_____	_____	_____
23	____	____	_____	_____	_____
24	____	____	_____	_____	_____
25	____	____	_____	_____	_____
26	____	____	_____	_____	_____
27	____	____	_____	_____	_____
28	____	____	_____	_____	_____
29	____	____	_____	_____	_____
30	____	____	_____	_____	_____
31	____	____	_____	_____	_____

	Responses Emotional	**Responses** Physical
1	_____	_____
2	_____	_____
3	_____	_____
4	_____	_____
5	_____	_____
6	_____	_____
7	_____	_____
8	_____	_____
9	_____	_____
10	_____	_____
11	_____	_____
12	_____	_____
13	_____	_____
14	_____	_____
15	_____	_____
16	_____	_____
17	_____	_____
18	_____	_____
19	_____	_____
20	_____	_____
21	_____	_____
22	_____	_____
23	_____	_____
24	_____	_____
25	_____	_____
26	_____	_____
27	_____	_____
28	_____	_____
29	_____	_____
30	_____	_____
31	_____	_____

Major Life Stress Evaluation

Check those life events that pertain to you. This will help you evaluate the level of major stress in your life.

_____ Death of spouse or close family member

_____ Divorce from spouse

_____ Legal separation from spouse

_____ Loss of job

_____ Radical loss of financial security

_____ Major personal injury or illness (gynecological or other cause)

_____ Future surgery for gynecological or other illness

_____ Beginning a new marriage

_____ Foreclosure of mortgage or loan

_____ Lawsuit lodged against you

_____ Marriage reconciliation

_____ Change in health of a family member

_____ Major trouble with boss or co-workers

_____ Increase in responsibility—job or home

_____ Learning you are pregnant

_____ Difficulties with your sexual abilities

_____ Gaining a new family member

_____ Change to a different job

_____ Increase in number of marital arguments

_____ New loan or mortgage

_____ Son or daughter leaving home

_____ Major disagreement with in-laws or friends

_____ Spouse beginning or stopping work

_____ Recognition for outstanding achievements

_____ Beginning or ending education

_____ Undergoing a change in living conditions

___ Revising or altering your personal habits

___ Change in work hours or conditions

___ Change of residence

___ Change in school or major

___ Alterations in your recreational activities

___ Change in church or club activities

___ Change in social activities

___ Change in sleeping habits

___ Change in number of family get-togethers

___ Change in diet or eating habits

___ Going on vacation

___ Occurrence of the year-end holidays

___ Committing a minor violation of the law

Key to Major Life Stress and Anxiety

Major life stress can have a significant impact on the emotional symptoms of anxiety and nervous tension as well as on other health problems linked to these symptoms. It is helpful to assess your own level of stress to see how it may be impacting your health. One popular tool is the Holmes and Rahe Social Readjustment Rating Scale, first published in 1967. The scale above is adapted for women and identifies events that cause stress.

Checking many items in the first third of this scale indicates major life stress and a possible vulnerability to serious illness. As you go down the list, the stresses decrease in the degree to which they cause major emotional dislocation. For example, a death or divorce is much more traumatic for most people than changing their school or major. Thus, the more items checked in the first two-thirds of the scale, the higher your stress quotient. Do everything possible to manage your stress in a healthy way. Eat the foods that provide a high-nutrient/low-stress diet, exercise on a regular basis, and learn the methods for managing stress given in Chapters 6 and 7 on stress reduction and deep breathing.

If you check fewer items, you are probably at lower risk for illness. Because stresses too minimal to include in this evaluation may also play a part in increasing your level of anxiety and nervous tension, you will still benefit from practicing the methods outlined in the chapter on stress reduction. Stress management is very important in helping you gain control over your level of muscle tension.

Daily Stress Evaluation

Check each item that seems to apply to you.

Work

____ Too much responsibility. You feel you have to push too hard to do your work. There are too many demands made of you. You feel pressured by all this responsibility. You worry about getting all your work done and doing it well.

____ Time urgency. You worry about getting your work done on time. You always feel rushed, and feel like there are not enough hours in the day to complete your work.

____ Job instability. You are concerned about losing your job. There are layoffs at your company. There is much insecurity and concern among your fellow employees about their job security.

____ Job performance. You don't feel that you are working up to your maximum capability because of outside pressures or stress. You are unhappy with your job performance and concerned about job security as a result.

____ Difficulty getting along with co-workers and boss. Your boss is too picky and critical. Your boss demands too much. You must work closely with co-workers who are difficult to get along with.

____ Uncomfortable physical plant. Lights are too bright or too dim; noises are too loud. You're exposed to noxious fumes or chemicals. There is too much activity going on around you, making it difficult to concentrate.

Home

____ Home organization. Home is poorly organized. It always seems messy; chores are half-finished. You feel tense and stressed while in your own home due to the physical disorder.

____ Time. There is too much to do in the home and never enough time to get it all done.

____ Too much responsibility. You need more help. There are too many demands on your time and energy. You feel tense and anxious as a result

Spouse or Significant Other

____ Hostile communication. There is too much negative emotion and drama. You are always upset and angry. There is not enough peace and quiet.

____ Not enough communication. There is not enough discussion of feelings or issues. You tend to hold in your feelings, which creates a strong feeling of bottled-up tension and stress.

____ Discrepancy in communication. One person talks about feelings too much, the other person too little.

____ Affection. Intimacy issues make you feel anxious and upset. There is a discrepancy between your needs in a relationship and what you receive from your partner. Either you feel you do not receive enough affection, or you are made uncomfortable by your partner's demands.

___ Sexuality. Sexual issues cause you to feel anxious and upset. There is a demand for too-frequent sexual relations by your partner. You feel pressured. Or you feel irritable, angry, and stressed because of a lack of sexual intimacy. You feel deprived by your partner.

___ Children. They make too much noise. They make too many demands on your time. They are hard to discipline. You find that dealing with your children increases your level of anxiety.

___ Extended family (parents, siblings, other relatives). Family relationships create anxiety and stress. Family members are negative, critical, or demanding; they engage in inappropriate social behavior or addictive behavior. Communications from family or interaction with family triggers negative emotional response.

Your Emotional State

___ Too much negative self-talk. You worry too much about every little thing. You constantly worry about what can go wrong in your life.

___ Excessive fearfulness of situations. You are fearful of being in certain situations or locations, such as going into an elevator, visiting a shopping mall, eating in restaurants, or going to a dental or doctor appointment.

___ Excessive fearfulness of public activities. You are afraid of public speaking, sitting in a social or work group, or going to parties or receptions.

___ Victimization. You experience that everyone is taking advantage of you or wants to hurt you.

___ Poor self-image. You don't like yourself enough. You are always finding fault with yourself.

_____ Too critical. You are always finding fault with others. You always look at what is wrong with other people rather than seeing their virtues.

_____ Inability to relax. You are always wound up. It is difficult for you to relax. You are tense and restless.

_____ Not enough self-renewal. You don't play enough or take enough time off to relax and have fun. As a result, life isn't fun and enjoyable.

_____ Feelings of depression. Feelings of depression alternate with anxiety. During your down times, you feel blue, isolated, and tearful. You feel a sense of self-blame and hopelessness. Fatigue and low-energy are problems.

_____ Too angry. Small life issues seem to upset you unduly. You find yourself becoming angry and irritable with your husband, children, or clients.

Key to Daily Stress Evaluation

This evaluation is very important for women with anxiety. Not all stresses have a major impact in our lives, like death, divorce, or personal injury. Most of us are exposed to a multitude of small life stresses on a daily basis. In some women with excessive anxiety and nervous tension, these stresses can trigger major episodes of emotional upset. In addition, the effects of these stresses can be cumulative. They can be a major factor in creating chronic wear and tear on our immune system, endocrine system, and circulatory system. And daily stress often triggers chronic muscle tension and pain.

Read over the day-to-day stress areas that you find difficult to handle. Becoming aware of them is the first step toward lessening their effects on your life. Methods for reducing them and helping your body to deal with them are given in Chapters 6, 7, 9, and 10 on stress reduction, breathing exercises, yoga, and acupressure.

Finding the Solution

3

Dietary Principles for Relief of Anxiety & Stress

Many women are unaware of the important role that food selection can play in either intensifying or reducing symptoms of anxiety, panic, and excessive stress. Medical research in the areas of diet and nutrition over the past 20 years has shown that many foods, beverages, and food additives can worsen or trigger anxiety feelings in women. This is true in emotionally based as well as chemically or hormonally based cases of anxiety and panic. In contrast, studies have found certain foods to be beneficial for their mood-stabilizing and calming properties.

In my practice, I have been impressed by the importance of an antianxiety diet. I have seen thousands of women, suffering anxiety symptoms due to many different emotional and physical causes, improve when they change their diets. Diet can be the primary treatment for anxiety caused by PMS, hypoglycemia, and food allergies; the use of an antianxiety diet can play a major supporting role in reducing unpleasant stress symptoms. In fact, I have found that continuing stressful eating habits works against other therapeutic measures a patient may institute, such as counseling or the use of antianxiety medication. Thus, the importance of healthful dietary practices in the treatment of anxiety should not be underestimated.

In this chapter, I list and discuss in detail the foods that worsen anxiety and should be avoided. The list may surprise you because it contains not only processed "junk food," but also foods that are considered staples of the American diet. Many women with anxiety unwittingly eat a diet that worsens their symptoms. I also discuss foods that can improve and enhance your emotional well-being as well as your general state of health. This information is based on extensive work with women who suffered from fatigue and noted significant relief of their symptoms when following this program. It is also based on the available medical research.

Foods to Avoid

It is important to eliminate all foods that intensify your anxiety symptoms. These include foods that are toxic and stressful to the body when used in excess, and that may trigger anxiety symptoms in susceptible women when used even in small amounts. In my experience with patients suffering from moderate to severe anxiety, all of these foods should be entirely eliminated or at least sharply curtailed to small amounts, used on an occasional basis as a treat. Some women may find that they need to eliminate anxiety-causing foods gradually because of their emotional or physical attachments to the food. When there are strong emotional attachments, the elimination process itself can cause stress; thus, it should be done gently. Many other women find that the "cold turkey" approach works best, and they appreciate the rapid relief from anxiety symptoms that simply eliminating a stressful food brings. I will mention any pitfalls of such an approach when discussing the specific foods in this section.

Caffeine. Coffee, black tea, soft drinks, and chocolate all contain caffeine. Many women with anxiety and high levels of stress mistakenly use caffeine as a pick-me-up to help them get through the day's tasks. Unfortunately, caffeine can trigger and aggravate anxiety and panic episodes. Caffeine used in excess (more than four or five cups per day) can dramatically increase anxiety, irritability, and mood swings. Even small amounts can make susceptible women jittery. After the initial pick-up, women with anxiety coexisting with excessive stress find that caffeine intake makes them more tired than before.

Caffeine triggers anxiety and panic symptoms because it directly stimulates several arousal mechanisms in the body. It increases the brain's level of norepinephrine, a neurotransmitter that increases alertness. However, it also triggers sympathetic nervous system activity, which causes the fight-or-flight physiological responses in the body, such as increased pulse, breathing rate, and muscle tension. Thus, caffeine intake triggers the physiological responses typical of anxiety states. Also, caffeine stimulates the release of stress hormones from the adrenal glands, further intensifying symptoms of nervousness and jitteriness.

Caffeine depletes the body's stores of B-complex vitamins and essential minerals, such as potassium, which are important in the chemical reactions that convert food to usable energy. Deficiency of these nutrients increases anxiety, mood swings, and fatigue. Depletion of B-complex vitamins also interferes with carbohydrate metabolism and healthy liver function, which help to regulate the blood sugar as well as estrogen levels. An imbalance in estrogen and progesterone can increase anxiety and mood swings in women with symptoms of PMS or menopause. Many menopausal women also complain that caffeine increases the frequency of hot flashes. Coffee, black tea, chocolate, and soft drinks all act to inhibit iron absorption, thus worsening anemia.

If you suffer from moderate to severe anxiety symptoms due to any cause, I recommend that you reduce your caffeine consumption to one cup of coffee per day and try to eliminate cola drinks, caffeine-containing tea, and chocolate. Some women may find that going "cold turkey" with coffee and eliminating it abruptly causes unpleasant withdrawal symptoms such as headaches, depression, and fatigue. In these cases, it is better to cut down coffee intake gradually, decreasing the amounts slowly over a period of one month to several months, substituting first decaffeinated coffee and finally herbal teas. Many herbal teas, like chamomile, hops, and peppermint, even have a relaxant effect on the body, thereby helping to reduce anxiety.

Caffeine Content of Beverages and Foods

(listed in order of caffeine content)

Product	*Caffeine per Serving*
Coffee (per cup)	
Drip (average)	146 mg
Percolated (average)	110 mg
Coffee—instant (per cup)	
Folgers™	97.5 mg
Maxwell House™	94 mg
Nescafe™	81
Decaffeinated Coffee (per cup)	
Sanka™	4 mg
Brim™	3.5 mg
Taster's Choice™	3.5 mg
Tea (per cup)	
Tetley™	63.5 mg
Lipton™	52 mg
Constant Comment™	29 mg
Soft Drinks (per 12 oz. can)	
Tab™	56.6 mg
Mountain Dew™	55 mg
Diet Dr. Pepper™	54 mg
Coke Classic™	46 mg
Diet Coke™	46 mg
Pepsi™	38.4 mg
Diet Pepsi™	36 mg
Hot Chocolate Drinks (per cup)	
Cocoa	13 mg
Candy (per oz.)	
Ghirardelli™ Dark Chocolate	24 mg
Hershey's™ Milk Chocolate	4 mg

Sugar. Glucose, a simple form of sugar, is the food that provides the body with its main source of energy. Without a steady supply of glucose, we could not produce the hundreds of thousands of chemical reactions our bodies need to perform daily functions. The brain is one of the primary users of glucose, requiring 20 percent of the total available glucose to function optimally. However, the form in which you take this important food into your body can affect your mood in a profound manner. The ideal approach is to eat lots of complex carbohydrates such as whole grains, potatoes, fruit, and vegetables. The sugar in these foods digests slowly and is released into the blood circulation very gradually. Thus, the amount of sugar released from these foods does not overwhelm the body's ability to handle it.

Unfortunately, many Americans obtain their sugar intake through the excessive use of simple sugar—the refined white or brown sugar that is the primary ingredient of most cookies, candies, cakes, pies, soft drinks, ice cream, and other sweet foods. In addition, pasta and bread made from white flour, which has all the bran, essential fatty acids, and nutrients removed, act as simple sugars; unfortunately, these make up a significant part of the diet of many women in Western societies. Many convenience foods, including salad dressing, catsup, and relish, also contain high levels of both sugar and salt. With sugar so prevalent in many foods, sugar addiction is common in our society among people of all ages. Many people use sweet foods as a way to deal with their frustrations and other upsets. As a result, most Americans consume too much sugar—the average American eats 120 pounds per year.

This excessive level of sugar intake can be a major trigger for anxiety symptoms. Here is what happens: Unlike complex carbohydrates, foods based on sugar and white flour break down quickly in the digestive tract. Glucose is released rapidly into the blood circulation and from there is absorbed by the cells of the body to satisfy their energy needs. To handle this overload, the pancreas must release large amounts of insulin, a chemical that helps move the glucose from the blood circulation into the cells.

Often the pancreas tends to overshoot the amount of insulin needed. As a result, the blood sugar level goes from too high to too low, resulting in the roller coaster effect typically seen in hypoglycemia or PMS. You may initially feel "high" after eating sugar, and then experience a rapid crash and a dip in your energy level. (Excessive amounts of stress also use up glucose rapidly and can cause similar symptoms.) When your blood sugar level falls too low, you begin to feel anxious, jittery, spacey, and confused because your brain is deprived of its necessary fuel. To remedy this situation, the adrenal glands release cortisol and other hormones that cause your liver to release stored sugar so that your blood sugar can return to normal levels. Though the adrenal hormones boost the blood sugar level, they unfortunately increase arousal symptoms and anxiety too. Thus, both the initial glucose deprivation in the brain and the adrenal's response to restore the glucose levels can intensify symptoms of anxiety and panic in susceptible women.

Excessive use of sugar has further detrimental effects. Like caffeine, sugar depletes the body's B-complex vitamins and minerals, thereby increasing nervous tension, anxiety, and irritability. Too much sugar also intensifies fatigue by narrowing the diameter of the blood vessels and putting stress on the nervous system. Candida feeds on sugar, so overindulging in this high-stress food worsens chronic candida infections. Many women with chronic candida complain of emotional symptoms like depression and nervous tension. Furthermore, sugar (as well as caffeine, alcohol, flavor enhancers, and white flour) appears to be an important trigger for the binge eating often seen with anxiety and PMS. In fact, research studies have shown that when women switch from a diet high in sugar to a sugar-free, high-nutrient diet, food addictive behavior tends to cease. After making the switch from a high-sugar-intake diet, women tend to lose or maintain weight more easily and to successfully maintain relief from the pattern of craving and binging (for up to two years, in one study).

In summary, sugar stresses many bodily systems, worsens your health, and intensifies anxiety, nervous tension, and fatigue. Try to satisfy your sweet tooth instead with healthier foods. Consider fruit or grain-based desserts, like oatmeal cookies sweetened with fruit or honey. You will find that small amounts of these foods can satisfy your cravings. Instead of disrupting your mood and energy level, they actually have a healthful and balancing effect.

Alcohol. Women with moderate to severe anxiety and mood swings should avoid alcohol entirely or limit its use to occasional small amounts. Alcohol is a simple sugar, rapidly absorbed by the body. Like other sugars, alcohol increases hypoglycemia symptoms; excessive use can increase anxiety and mood swings. (See the preceding section on sugar for a thorough discussion of this process.) This can be particularly pronounced in women with PMS-related hypoglycemia.

Once alcohol has been absorbed and assimilated, it is primarily metabolized by the liver. This is a complex process requiring much work on the part of the body. Excessive intake of alcohol can overwhelm the liver's ability to process it, leading to toxic by-products that can themselves affect mood. Too much alcohol can also impede the body's ability to detoxify other chemicals—including drugs, hormones such as estrogen, and pesticides—that we take into our bodies by choice or through environmental contact. As a result, toxic levels of these chemicals can build up in the body, worsening anxiety. Excessive levels of estrogen seen in women with PMS, young women on birth control pills, and menopausal women on estrogen replacement therapy, have been linked to altered mood states and anxiety. This can occur when the therapeutic estrogen dose prescribed by the physician is in excess of the body's needs.

Alcohol, an irritant to the liver as well as to other parts of the digestive tract, may be used by the body for immediate energy or stored in the liver or in the rest of the body as fat. Unfortunately, the liver cannot convert alcohol to a storage form of glucose. As a result, the amount of fat stored in the liver increases with excessive alcohol use. Alcohol raises the liver enzyme level, leading to liver inflammation (or hepatitis). Eventually the chemical by-products of alcohol and the fat derived from alcohol can cause scarring and shrinkage of the liver, leading to functional impairment of the liver and cirrhosis. In addition, alcohol irritates the lining of the upper digestive tract, including the esophagus, stomach, and upper part of the small intestine. It also causes irritation and inflammation of the pancreas. Over time, this can result in worsening of hypoglycemia and diabetes as well as impaired absorption and assimilation of essential nutrients from the small intestine. Certain of these nutrients, such as the B vitamins, are necessary to stabilize these conditions.

The nervous system is particularly susceptible to the deleterious effects of alcohol, which readily crosses the blood-brain barrier and actually destroys brain cells. Alcohol can cause profound behavioral and psychological changes in women who use it excessively. Symptoms include emotional upset, irrational anger, emotional outbursts, poor judgment, loss of memory, mental impairment, dizziness, poor coordination, and difficulty in walking.

Symptoms of emotional upset triggered by alcohol can also be caused by candida overgrowth, since candida thrive on the sugar in alcohol. Alcohol can thus promote a tendency toward chronic candida infections. Women with candida-related mood upset and fatigue need to avoid alcohol entirely. Furthermore, many women with allergies are sensitive to the yeast in alcohol, which worsens their allergic symptoms.

Given the preceding information on alcohol's adverse effects, I recommend that women with anxiety symptoms use alcohol only very rarely. When used carefully—not exceeding 4 ounces of wine per day, 12 ounces of beer, or 1 ounce of hard liquor—alcohol can have a delightfully relaxing effect in women who have normal energy levels. It can make us more sociable and enhance the taste of food. However, women who are particularly susceptible to the negative effects of alcohol shouldn't drink at all. If you entertain a great deal and enjoy social drinking, try nonalcoholic beverages. A nonalcoholic cocktail, such as mineral water with a twist of lime or lemon or a dash of bitters, is a good substitute. "Near beer" is a nonalcoholic beer substitute that tastes quite good. Light wine and beer have a lower alcohol content than hard liquor, liqueurs, and regular wine.

Food Additives. Several thousand chemical additives are currently used in commercial food manufacturing. Some of the most popular, including aspartame (Nutrasweet™), monosodium glutamate (MSG), nitrates, and nitrites, produce allergic and anxiety-like symptoms in many people. I have had patients complain that the use of the artificial sweetener aspartame precipitated panic-like symptoms, such as rapid heartbeat, shallow breathing, headaches, anxiety, spaciness, and dizziness. Since aspartame is used in so many processed diet foods, susceptible women may need to avoid low-calorie, sugar-free drinks, jams, desserts, and other foods. If you are susceptible to aspartame, be sure to carefully read the labels of any processed diet foods before you buy them.

Many woman are also very susceptible to the chemical MSG, a flavor enhancer that is often used in food preparation in Chinese restaurants. MSG causes headaches and anxiety episodes in some people, and patients have also reported that this chemical increased their food cravings and food addictions. If you are sensitive to MSG, check labels of bottled dressing and sauces to make sure that it is not an ingredient. Also, eat at Chinese restaurants that advertise "NO MSG." Many restaurants are aware of the common sensitivity to MSG and forgo using it in their food preparation.

Nitrates and nitrites can produce allergies also. These chemicals are used as preservatives in many foods, especially cured meats such as hot dogs, bacon, and ham. Be sure to check the labels on foods that you suspect might contain nitrates or nitrites if you are sensitive to these chemicals.

Dairy Products. Women with anxiety and stress symptoms should avoid dairy products. This always surprises women, because dairy products have traditionally been touted as one of the four basic food groups; many women count them as staples in their diet, eating large amounts of cheese, yogurt, milk, and cottage cheese. Yet dairy products are extremely difficult for the body to digest; they can worsen the depression and fatigue that coexist in many women with anxiety symptoms. This is because the body must use so much energy to break them down before they can be absorbed, assimilated, and finally utilized. All parts of dairy products are difficult to digest—the fat, the protein, and the milk sugar. Digesting dairy products demands hydrochloric acids, enzymes, and fat emulsifiers, which a stressed and tired woman may not produce in sufficient quantities.

Many women are specifically allergic to dairy products, and dairy products intensify allergy symptoms in general. Besides physical symptoms, food allergies can trigger anxiety, mood swings, and even fatigue in susceptible women. I see this often in my patients who have emotionally-based anxiety symptoms or PMS-related anxiety coexisting with food allergies. Users of dairy products often complain of allergy-based nasal congestion, sinus swelling, and postnasal drip. They can also suffer from digestive problems such as bloating, gas, and bowel changes, which intensify with menstruation. Intolerance to dairy products can hamper the absorption and assimilation of calcium, an important anxiety-relieving mineral.

Dairy products have many other unhealthy effects on a woman's body. The saturated fats in dairy products put women at higher risk of heart disease and cancer of the breast, uterus, and ovaries. Women on a high-fat diet also tend to accumulate excess weight more easily. Many dairy products, such as cheese, are high in salt as well as fat. Excessive use of these foods can increase the risk of high blood pressure and of bloating and fluid retention. Bloating can cause uncomfortable breast tenderness and abdominal swelling, particularly in the premenstrual period.

Women who have depended on dairy products for their calcium intake naturally wonder what alternative sources they should use. Women concerned about calcium intake can turn to many other good dietary sources of this essential nutrient, including beans, peas, soybeans, sesame seeds, soup stock made from chicken or fish bones, and green leafy vegetables. For food preparation, soy milk, potato milk, and nut milk are excellent substitutes. These nondairy milks are readily available at health food stores. You can also use a supplement containing calcium, magnesium, and vitamin D to make sure your intake is sufficient.

Red Meats and Poultry. Like dairy products, meat tends to increase depression and fatigue because it is difficult for the body to digest. Because of the extremely tough quality of the protein in meat, as well as the high content of saturated fats, the body must work hard to reduce the protein to amino acids and the saturated fats to fatty acids. However, if you need to include meat in your diet, chicken with the skin removed may be a better choice than red meat because it is lower in saturated fat content. Many women with anxiety coexisting with depression and chronic fatigue feel exhausted after a heavy meal of meat. Meat intake can worsen mood symptoms and fatigue in other ways. The body uses the saturated fats in meat (and dairy products) to produce a group of hormones called the series-two prostaglandins. These hormones, found in tissues throughout the body, have negative health effects. They cause contraction of muscles and blood vessels and thereby increase cramps, PMS, high blood pressure, and irritable bowel syndrome. These hormones also put stress on the immune function and trigger inflammation. As a result, they can worsen infections of all types, decrease resistance, and trigger allergy symptoms. Eating meat with high saturated-fat content as a major part of the diet, like eating dairy products, puts women at risk for heart disease, breast cancer, cancer of the reproductive tract, and obesity.

If you have anxiety or excessive stress in your life, you should sharply curtail your meat consumption. Obtain your protein from vegetable sources, such as legumes, starches, raw seeds, and grains. You may eat fish occasionally, too. Fish has the added benefit of containing high levels of the beneficial essential fatty acids that improve vitality.

Wheat and Other Gluten-containing Grains. Women who have food allergies or PMS- or menopause-related mood problems may have difficulty digesting wheat. The protein in wheat, called gluten, is highly allergenic and difficult for the body to break down, absorb, and assimilate. Women with wheat intolerance are prone to fatigue, depression, bloating, intestinal gas, and bowel changes.

In my clinical experience, wheat consumption by anxious and depressed women who are nutritionally sensitive can worsen emotional symptoms and fatigue. I have seen this happen with patients during the week or two before the onset of menses. Many menopausal women tolerate wheat poorly because their digestive tracts are beginning to show the wear and tear of aging and don't produce enough enzymes to handle wheat easily.

Women with allergies often find that wheat intensifies nasal and sinus congestion as well as fatigue. I also find that women with poor resistance and a tendency toward infections may need to eliminate wheat in order to boost their immune function. Because wheat is leavened with yeast, it should be also avoided by women with candida infections.

No matter what the cause of your anxiety, if the symptoms are severe, you should probably eliminate wheat from your diet at least for one to three months during the early stages of recovery. Oats and rye, which also contain gluten, should be eliminated initially along with wheat. Many allergic and severely upset and fatigued women don't even handle corn or rice well. Although these do not contain gluten, most women use them so frequently that they build up an intolerance during times of fatigue.

I have found over the years that the least stressful grain for severely stressed women is buckwheat, probably because it is not commonly eaten in our society. Also, it is not in the same plant family as wheat and other grains. Other infrequently used grains such as quinoa and amaranth may be tried as well. These are the grain base of many pastas and cereals available in health food stores. As women with anxiety start to regain their emotional equilibrium, they may add rice and corn back into the diet, still eliminating wheat, oats, and rye until their recovery is complete. Women with milder to moderate symptoms of anxiety may want to keep rice and corn in their diet but still look for the benefits of a trial of wheat elimination.

Salt. Although salt does not specifically increase anxiety, women should watch their salt intake carefully and avoid excessive intake for optimal health and well-being. Too much salt in the diet can cause many physical problems. It can worsen bloating and fluid retention, as well as increase high blood pressure, and is a risk factor in the development of osteoporosis in menopausal women. In addition, salt can deplete the body of potassium, a mineral necessary for healthy nervous system function.

Unfortunately, most processed foods contain large amounts of salt. Frozen and canned foods are often loaded with salt. In fact, one frozen-food entree can contribute as much as one-half teaspoon of salt to your daily intake. Large amounts of salt are also commonly found in the American diet as table salt (sodium chloride), MSG (monosodium glutamate), and a variety of food additives. Fast foods such as hamburgers, hot dogs, french fries, pizza, and tacos are loaded with salt and saturated fats. Common processed foods such as soups, potato chips, cheese, olives, salad dressings, and catsup (to name only a few) are also very high in salt. To make matters worse, many people use too much salt while cooking and seasoning their meals.

For women of all ages, I recommend eliminating added salt in your meals. For flavor, use seasonings such as garlic, herbs, spices, and lemon juice. Avoid processed foods that are high in salt, including canned foods, olives, pickles, potato chips, tortilla chips, catsup, and salad dressings. Learn to read labels and look for the word *sodium* (salt). If it appears high on the list of ingredients, don't buy the product. Many items in health food stores are labeled "no salt added." Some supermarkets offer "no added salt" foods in their diet or health food sections.

Summary Chart: Foods to Avoid

Coffee
Tea (containing caffeine)
Chocolate
Cola drinks
Other soft drinks containing caffeine
Sugar
Alcohol

    Foods and beverages flavored with aspartame *(Nutrasweet™)* or *monosodium glutamate (MSG)*

Dairy products
Red meat, poultry
Wheat, oats, rye
Salt

Foods That Help Relieve Anxiety

The foods you should eat when anxious, depressed, or fatigued should leave you feeling as good as, or better than, you felt before the meal. These foods should also support and accelerate the healing process of the illness that underlies the emotional symptoms. To achieve these goals means initially limiting your diet to low-stress foods. As your anxiety symptoms diminish, you can eat a wider range of foods. Begin to develop an awareness of how your food selections affect your emotional well-being. If a particular food makes you feel anxious, jittery, depressed, or fatigued when you eat it, you should eliminate it.

I have found that certain groups of foods are tolerated by nearly everyone, even women who are anxious and upset. These foods include most vegetables, fruits, starches, a few grains such as buckwheat, quinoa, amaranth, corn, and rice (in women who do not have severe PMS or food allergies), and nuts. Initially, these should be your core food selection. As you feel better, you can add more fruits, grains, oils, fish, and poultry (in moderation).

In this section I describe the antianxiety and mood-stabilizing effects of these beneficial foods.

Vegetables. These are outstanding foods for the relief of stress. Many vegetables are high in calcium, magnesium, and potassium—important minerals that help improve stamina, endurance, and vitality. Both magnesium and potassium, used in supplemental form in clinical studies, have been shown to reduce depression and increase energy levels dramatically. For women who suffer from tension and anxiety, the essential minerals in vegetables have a relaxant effect, relieving muscular tension and calming the emotions. Both calcium and magnesium act as natural tranquilizers, a real benefit for women suffering from stress and upset. The potassium content of vegetables helps relieve congestive symptoms by reducing fluid retention and bloating. Some of the best sources for these minerals include Swiss chard, spinach, broccoli, beet greens, mustard greens, and kale.

Many vegetables are high in vitamin C, which helps strengthen capillaries, thereby facilitating the flow of essential nutrients throughout the body, as well as the flow of waste products out. Vitamin C is also an important antistress vitamin because it promotes healthy adrenal hormone production (the adrenal glands help us deal with stress). This is particularly important for women with anxiety caused by emotional upset, allergies, or stress from other origins, such as the environment. Vitamin C is also important for immune function and wound healing. Its anti-infectious properties may help reduce the tendency toward respiratory, bladder, and vaginal infections. Vegetables high in vitamin C include brussels sprouts, broccoli, cauliflower, kale, peppers, parsley, peas, tomatoes, and potatoes.

Carrots, spinach, squash, turnip greens, collards, parsley, green onions, and kale are among the vegetables highest in vitamin A. Vitamin A strengthens the cell walls and protects the mucous membranes. This helps protect you from respiratory disease as well as allergic episodes. Vitamin A is important for women with anxiety whose resistance is low and who are thus prone to allergies and infections. Vitamin A deficiency has been linked to fatigue as well as night blindness, skin aging, loss of smell, loss of appetite, and softening of bones and teeth. Luckily, it is easy to get an abundance of vitamin A from vegetables.

Vegetables are composed primarily of water and carbohydrates. Because they contain very little protein and fat, they tend to be easy to digest. However, some women find that they have fewer digestive problems with cooked vegetables. Cooking breaks down and softens the fiber in the vegetables, making less work for the body in the digestion process. Steaming is the best cooking method, because it preserves the essential nutrients. Some women with extreme stress and fatigue may even want to puree their vegetables in a blender. As you begin to recover your emotional balance and energy level, I recommend adding raw foods such as salads, vegetable juices, and raw vegetables to your meals for more texture and variety.

Fruits. Fruits also contain a wide range of nutrients that can relieve anxiety and stress. Like many vegetables, fruits are an excellent source of vitamin C, which is important for healthy blood vessels and blood circulation, as well as for antistress and immune-stimulant properties. Almost all fruits contain some vitamin C, the best sources being berries and melons. These fruits are also good sources of bioflavonoids, another essential nutrient that affects blood vessel strength and permeability. Bioflavonoids also have an anti-inflammatory effect, important to women with allergies, menstrual cramps, or arthritis. Bioflavonoids are supportive of the female reproductive tract and can improve mood and increase energy levels. Although citrus fruits (oranges, grapefruits) are excellent sources of bioflavonoids and vitamin C, they are highly acidic and difficult for many women with food allergies or sensitive digestive tracts to digest; therefore, such women should avoid them in the early stages of treatment.

Certain fruits—including raisins, blackberries, and bananas—are excellent sources of calcium and magnesium, two essential minerals for proper nervous system and muscular function. Raisins and bananas are also exceptional sources of potassium, good for women with excessive fatigue and bloating. All fruits, in fact, are excellent sources of potassium.

Eat fruits whole to benefit from their high fiber content, which helps prevent constipation and other digestive irregularities. For snacks and desserts, fresh fruits are excellent substitutes for cookies, candies, cakes, and other foods high in refined sugar. Although fruit is high in sugar, its high fiber content helps slow down absorption of the sugar into the blood circulation and thereby helps stabilize the blood sugar level. I recommend, however, that women with anxiety and stress do not consume fruit juices. Fruit juice does not contain the bulk or fiber of the whole fruit. As a result, it acts more like table sugar and can destabilize your blood sugar level dramatically when used to excess. This can exacerbate anxiety, fatigue, and mood swings.

Starches. Potatoes, sweet potatoes, and yams are soft, well-tolerated carbohydrates that provide an additional source of easy-to-digest protein for women with anxiety and nervous tension. Like the other complex carbohydrates, starches calm the mood by helping to regulate the blood sugar level. You can steam, mash, bake, and eat them alone, or include them in other low-stress dishes and casseroles. Starches combine very well with a variety of vegetables and can form the basis of delicious, low-stress meals. You can also combine them with lentils or split peas in soup.

Potatoes, especially sweet potatoes, are an exceptional source of vitamin A, so they can help boost resistance to infections and allergies. Potatoes and yams are also good sources of vitamin C and several of the B vitamins that help women handle anxiety and stress better and reduce fatigue.

Legumes. Beans and peas are excellent sources of calcium, magnesium, and potassium, which are necessary for healthy nervous system function, as well as for their emotional and muscle-relaxant properties. I highly recommend their use in a diet to combat depression and fatigue. Legumes are also very high in vitamin B complex and vitamin B_6, necessary nutrients for the relief and prevention of anxiety, menstrual fatigue, PMS symptoms, and cramps. They are also excellent sources of protein and, when eaten with grains, provide all the essential amino acids. (Good examples of low-stress grain and legume combinations include meals of beans and buckwheat, or corn bread and split pea soup.) Legumes provide an excellent, easily utilized source of protein and can be substituted for meat at many meals.

Legumes are an excellent source of fiber that can help normalize bowel function. They digest slowly and can help to regulate the blood sugar level, a trait they share with whole grains. As a result, legumes are an ideal food for women with blood sugar imbalances caused by diabetes, anxiety, nervous tension, and diet.

Some women find gas to be a problem when they eat beans. You can minimize gas by taking digestive enzymes and eating beans in small quantities. Also, because legumes contain high levels of protein, women with severe fatigue or digestive problems may find them difficult to digest at first. For easier digestibility, I recommend beginning with green beans, green peas, split peas, lentils, lima beans, fresh sprouts, and possibly tofu (if you handle soy products well). As your energy level improves, add such delicious legumes as black beans, pinto beans, kidney beans, and chickpeas. These foods are high in iron and tend to be good sources of copper and zinc.

Whole Grains. Although you should eliminate some grains from your diet (especially wheat and other gluten-containing grains) when first starting an antianxiety program, many whole grains have tremendous health benefits for women suffering from nervous tension. Whole grains are excellent sources of mood-stabilizing nutrients like vitamin B complex, vitamin E, many essential minerals, complex carbohydrates, protein, essential fatty acids, and fiber. Like legumes, whole grains help stabilize the blood sugar level to prevent hypoglycemia-triggered anxiety symptoms.

Brown rice and corn are good choices for women with mild to moderate anxiety symptoms, as are buckwheat and more exotic grain alternatives, such as quinoa and amaranth. Pasta, cereals, flour, and other foods made from these grain alternatives can be purchased in health food stores.

Women with allergy-related anxiety symptoms need to be careful not to overdose on any one grain. Rotating a variety of nongluten-containing grains in the diet can prevent anxiety caused by allergic reactions or fatigue. Besides eating corn and rice as primary grains, you can find pasta and noodles, as well as flour for baking, made from these grains. Use corn tortillas instead of those made of wheat.

Seeds and Nuts.   Seeds and nuts are the best sources of the two essential fatty acids, linoleic acid and linolenic acid. These fatty acids provide the raw materials your body needs to produce the beneficial prostaglandin hormones. Adequate levels of essential fatty acids in your diet are very important in preventing both the emotional and physical symptoms of PMS, menopause, emotional upsets, and allergies. The best sources of both fatty acids are raw flax and pumpkin seeds. Other seeds, such as sesame and sunflower seeds, are excellent sources of linoleic acid. Seeds and nuts are also good sources of the B-complex vitamins and vitamin E, both of which are important antistress factors for women with muscle tension and emotional stress symptoms. These nutrients also help regulate hormonal balance. Like vegetables, seeds and nuts are very high in the essential minerals such as magnesium, calcium, and potassium needed by women with excessive muscle tension and emotional stress symptoms. Particularly beneficial are sesame seeds, sunflower seeds, pistachios, pecans, and almonds.

Nuts and seeds are very high in calories and can be difficult to digest, especially if they are roasted and salted. Therefore, you should eat them only in small to moderate amounts. Flax seed oil is one of the best sources of the essential fatty acids needed for production of the beneficial prostaglandin hormones. It has a rich, golden color and may be used as a butter substitute on vegetables, rice, potatoes, pasta, and popcorn. Unlike butter, flax oil cannot be used for cooking. Cook foods first; then add flax oil to the food for flavoring just before serving.

The oils in all seeds and nuts are very perishable, so avoid exposing them to light, heat, and oxygen. Refrigerate all shelled seeds and nuts as well as their oils to prevent rancidity. Try to eat them raw, and shell them yourself. Eating them raw and unsalted gives you the benefit of their essential fatty acids (beneficial for skin and hair), and you'll also avoid the negative effects of too much salt. Seeds and nuts make a wonderful garnish on salads, vegetable dishes, and casseroles. As your energy level improves, you can also eat them as a main source of protein in snacks and light meals.

Meat, Poultry, and Fish. I generally recommend eating meat only in small quantities or avoiding it altogether if you have moderate to severe anxiety. Red meats such as beef, pork, and lamb, as well as poultry, contain saturated fats and hard-to-digest protein. If you do want to eat meat, your best choice is fish. Unlike other meat, fish contains linolenic acid, one of the beneficial fatty acids that help relax your mood as well as your tense muscles. Fish is also an excellent source of minerals, especially iodine and potassium. Particularly good selections for women with anxiety are salmon, tuna, mackerel, and trout.

Most Americans eat much more protein than is healthy. Excessive amounts of protein are difficult to digest and stress the kidneys. If you do include meat in your anxiety program, use it in very small amounts (3 ounces or less per day). Instead of using meat as your only source of protein, increase your intake of grains, beans, raw seeds, and nuts, which contain not only protein but also many other important antianxiety nutrients. For many years I have recommended that my patients use meat mainly as a garnish and a flavoring for casseroles, stir-fries, and soups. I also suggest buying meat from organic, range-fed animals, because their exposure to pesticides, antibiotics, and hormones has been reduced. If you find meat difficult to digest, you may be deficient in hydrochloric acid. Try taking a small amount of hydrochloric acid with every meat-containing meal to see if your digestion improves.

4

Menus, Meal Plans & Recipes

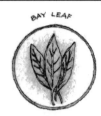

Once aware of the beneficial role that proper food selection can play in preventing and relieving anxiety and stress, a woman is usually quite motivated to shift her eating habits toward more healthy choices. Making the transition can present difficulties, however. Many of us tend to be creatures of habit, so the prospect of changing our food selection can appear difficult and intimidating. In addition, food fills emotional as well as nutritional needs for many women. For example, women commonly snack on "junk foods" like cookies, colas, candy bars, and other high-stress foods when they are feeling anxious. While these foods give an immediate emotional boost, the ingredients and additives contained in them often make the anxiety symptoms worse over time.

Over the years, my patients did best when I provided specific guidelines to help them through the transition period. When changing from a high-stress diet to an anxiety-relief food plan, my patients requested specific menus and meal plans. Although information on which foods to eat and which to avoid is tremendously helpful, most women want to know how to take the next step and combine the right foods in healthful meals. They also ask how to make the transition from their old diet to a new program without too much difficulty or confusion. Many of my patients benefited enormously from these simple and easy-to-follow guidelines, so I have included the information in this chapter for your benefit, too.

Before discussing the actual plans, I want to emphasize three principles that will make the transition process easier.

Make All Dietary Changes Gradually

Make the transition to a healthful anxiety-relief diet in an easy and nonstressful manner. Don't try to change all your dietary habits at once by making a clean sweep of your refrigerator and pantry. I've seen patients do that and come to my office in an absolute panic.

Instead, gradually substitute healthy foods for high-stress foods you have been eating. To do this, periodically review the lists of foods to limit and foods to emphasize. Each time you review this list, pick several foods that you are willing to eliminate and several to try. Review these lists as often as you choose, but do it on a regular basis. Every small change that you make in your diet can help.

Keep Your Meals Simple and Easy to Prepare

Many women lead busy, active lives and don't have a lot of time to cook complicated meals. For that reason, I've kept my meal plans quick and simple to prepare, with the main emphasis on foods that are delicious and high in nutrition. For those who are used to eating quick meals at fast-food restaurants or commercial snack food that is high in fat, sugar, and food additives, these simple meals offer a much healthier alternative.

Eat Smaller, More Frequent Meals or Snacks

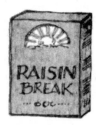

Women with anxiety symptoms feel better if they eat more frequently during the day. This helps stabilize the blood sugar level and reduce the "roller coaster" emotional and energetic highs and lows typical of PMS and hypoglycemia. If you don't want to actually eat smaller, more frequent meals, at least eat a healthful snack each period between meals to avoid symptoms of anxiety and jitteriness. Excellent snacks combine complex carbohydrates, protein, and essential fatty acids. Good examples include raw sunflower seeds or almonds, rice cakes with almond butter or tuna fish spread, air-popped popcorn, and fresh fruit such as apples, pears, and bananas.

Breakfast

Breakfast is actually the most important meal of the day. If breakfast foods containing complex carbohydrates, essential fatty acids, and protein are combined properly they help to calm your mood. They do this by stabilizing the blood sugar level and providing the body with many important nutrients for healthy nervous system function. Healthful and nourishing foods will provide the vigor and vitality you need to sail through your work and activities.

Unfortunately, many women skip breakfast entirely. This can worsen both the symptoms of anxiety and stress due to hypoglycemia, menopause, food allergies, and the anxiety episodes in women with mitral valve prolapse. Some women eat foods like doughnuts, sweet rolls, and coffee in hopes of getting quick energy, but these foods can instead increase nervous tension and anxiety. Others may eat hearty breakfasts full of high-stress foods—eggs, bacon, milk, toast, and butter. The high fat and salt content of these foods further stresses the body and impairs your health. Any one of these meals can wreak havoc for women.

The healthy breakfast plan includes beverage, fruit, and whole grain foods.

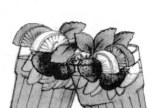

Beverages

The beverages you drink at breakfast can provide important nutrients and make you feel calm and relaxed throughout the day. Such beverages include herbal teas, roasted grain beverages (coffee substitutes), and nondairy milks. Good herbal teas for breakfast include chamomile and hops, which can calm your nerves if you tend to be anxious or edgy in the morning. Ginger is an excellent choice for women who tend to be tired in the morning and need a pick-me-up. Other healthful teas include blackberry, raspberry, and peppermint. Grain-based coffee substitutes such as Postum™, Pero™, or Cafix™ are hearty, satisfying beverages.

I strongly recommend that coffee drinkers switch to these beverages to avoid the stressful effects of caffeine. You can get the pick-me-up you're looking for, but in a much better way, through the use of proper herbs, vitamins and minerals, and exercise. Decaffeinated coffee in small amounts may be used as a transition beverage while making the switch to herbal teas or coffee substitutes.

Nondairy milk like soy, nut, or grain milk can be delicious, both as an occasional beverage or in cereal. Soy milk and potato-based milks are now easy to find in health food stores. You can make delicious nut milks easily and quickly in a blender (see Recipe section).

Women with anxiety and stress symptoms should use fruit juice cautiously. Fruit juice is a source of simple sugar, which can destabilize the blood sugar level and worsen anxiety, irritability, fatigue, and the inability to concentrate when used on a regular basis by susceptible women.

The most important drink of all is water, six to eight glasses per day. I recommend spring or filtered tap water. With the increasing pollution of our ground water, water purity is becoming a real health concern. Until this trend is reversed through adequate protection of our water supply, I recommend not drinking tap water if at all possible, or buying a filter for home use.

Fruits

Though fruit juice can worsen mood symptoms because of its concentrated sugar, whole fruits make a wonderful breakfast food. While fruits are high in sugar content, they are also high in fiber, which will make you feel full faster and decrease your appetite so that you don't overeat. The fiber in fruit also helps to regulate bowel function. Fruits are also great sources of such essential vitamins and minerals as vitamin C, vitamin A, and potassium.

In most areas a wide variety of fruits are available year-round, particularly apples, bananas, oranges, and grapefruit. These staples of the American diet are great breakfast foods. For nutritional variety, enjoy seasonal fruits such as apricots, peaches, berries, cherries, and melons. Whenever possible, eat locally grown fruits in season, as they will tend to be riper and fresher. Try to find unsprayed and organic fruit, to avoid pesticide exposure. Many supermarkets are beginning to carry unsprayed foods because of the consumer demand for clean products.

Whole Grain Foods

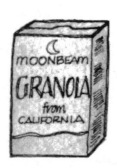

Whole grain-based foods are among the best breakfast foods for anxiety and stress. Whole grain foods are high in stress-combating vitamin B complex, magnesium, potassium, and vitamin E. They are high in complex carbohydrates, which are the best foods to stabilize your blood sugar and provide constant, slowly released energy throughout the day. Complex carbohydrates also help tremendously to normalize the mood swings and anxiety that some women suffer from during menopause or with PMS. These foods include the following:

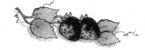

Hot Cereals. As I mentioned in the preceding chapter, rice, rye, and oats are preferable to wheat cereals for many women because of wheat's tendency to worsen depression and fatigue as well as allergies, bloating, and digestive upset. Your local health food store has a wide range of excellent grain cereals available. Look for cream of rye, cream of buckwheat, whole grain oatmeal, and seven- or four-grain cereals (without wheat). Choose brands with no added sugar. If there is no health food store near you, most supermarkets will have adequate products. I highly recommend Quaker™ whole oatmeal (not the quick-cooking refined product). Many of the "natural cereals" from the large companies are highly refined or highly sugared, so read labels carefully and watch out. Many supermarkets are beginning to carry bulk cereals in bins.

Cold Cereals. Health food stores carry a large number of whole-grain cold cereals, including puffed rice, corn, or millet, and unsweetened granola. At supermarkets, look for products that say "whole grain." Avoid cold cereals with added sugar.

I suggest moistening your cereal with nondairy milk: soy milk, nut milk, or the excellent new potato-based milks. Many of these are fortified with calcium, contain no saturated fat, and are digested relatively easily. Some women enjoy eating cold cereals dry or with a small amount of apple juice. For sweeteners, your best bet is fructose or maple syrup. They are very concentrated in flavor, so a little goes a long way.

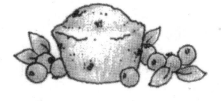

Muffins, Breads, and Crackers. A wide variety of grains can be found in the whole grain breads, muffins, and crackers now available in health food stores and supermarkets. There are also simple and easy-to-prepare recipes available if you wish to prepare baked goods such as oat muffins with extra oat bran, rye muffins, or corn bread. Rice cakes are commonly available at health food stores and now increasingly stocked at neighborhood supermarkets. You can also find wheat-free bread in health food stores. Muffins, bread, and crackers can be eaten with applesauce, nut butter, fruit, preserves, or a small amount of margarine. Try to avoid cow's milk butter, which is high in saturated fat.

Spreads. Almond butter and sesame butter (which are high in calcium) and soy spreads are good alternatives to cow's milk butter. Sesame butter is available in the foreign foods department of most supermarkets and can be found in health food stores. It is delicious as well as a wonderful source of nutrients. Sesame butter is also very filling, so a little goes a long way. I prefer buying the raw nut and seed butters rather than the toasted ones, as heating seeds and nuts alters the integrity of their fatty acids. (Fatty acids are used by the body to produce the beneficial relaxant prostaglandin hormones.) Applesauce and fruit preserves made without sugar are also good on toast, pancakes, and muffins.

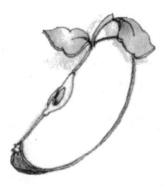

Breakfast Menus

The following easy-to-prepare menus provide a variety of healthful and delicious breakfast meals. They can also act as guidelines when you create your own meal plans. Recipes for the foods marked with an asterisk are included later in this chapter.

Bran muffin
Pear
Relaxant tea*

Oatmeal with maple syrup
Apple
Chamomile tea

Flax cereal with bananas*
Nondairy milk

Nondairy milk breakfast shake*
Bran muffin

Whole grain bread with
    raw almond butter
Fresh fruit preserves
Roasted grain beverage
    (coffee substitute)

High-protein flax shake*
Banana

Puffed rice cereal with berries
Nondairy milk

Tofu muesli cereal*
Peppermint tea

Cream of rye cereal with honey
Sunflower seeds
Orange

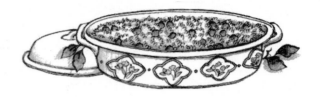

Lunch and Dinner

In their main meals, many women eat foods prepared with high-stress ingredients such as sugar, caffeine, and assorted flavorings that can actually increase anxiety and stress. In addition, many American lunches and dinners are higher in fat content (typically 30–40% saturated fat) than is good for general health and well-being. Lunches do not have to be rich and heavy affairs. In fact, lighter and more nutritious meals are preferable for women trying to recover from anxiety or stress-related problems. The following foods should be emphasized when planning your main meals of the day.

Soups

Soups are an excellent food for women with anxiety because they combine a variety of such highly nutritious ingredients as vegetables, grains, starches, legumes (beans and peas), and fish. These ingredients are good sources of vitamins, minerals, complex carbohydrates, and easy-to-digest protein that the cooking process helps to break down. Soups are also easy to prepare because you can combine the ingredients and then leave them to cook practically unattended while you do other things.

Homemade soups are recommend because you can avoid salt, high fat content, and food additives in the preparation. I have included several simple and delicious soup recipes. If you buy canned or powdered soup, use the "no added salt or sugar" types. Hain and Health Valley brands make soups labeled "no added salt," which are easy to find in health food stores. Read the soup product labels in your supermarket carefully.

Combining legume soup, such as lentil or split pea, with a grain product (cereal, toast) provides an excellent source of protein; grains and legumes complement each other in their amino acid content and together produce a high-quality protein.

You can increase the mineral content of the soup by combining a variety of vegetables that are high in potassium, calcium, and magnesium, such as carrots, turnips, and greens. The minerals tend to break out into the broth in the cooking process. You can boost the mineral content of your soup even further by adding chicken, fish, or bones to your soup base along with a few tablespoons of vinegar. The vinegar will pull calcium from the bones. This can help women who respond to the relaxant effect that calcium has on mood and muscle tension.

If you can't eat soup without some salt flavor, add one teaspoon of miso to your cup of soup. Miso is a fermented soy product of Japanese origin, easily found in Oriental markets and health food stores. It is much lower in salt content than regular table salt.

Salads

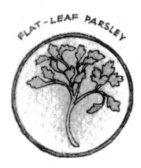

Women who are working to combat their anxiety or stress symptoms through nutrition often prefer to eat vegetables raw to protect their vitamin content (vitamins can be lost through cooking). Salads are a great way to do this since there are so many ways to combine raw vegetables in a tasty format.

Many greens are high in magnesium, calcium, and iron; beans are high in calcium. The more adventuresome you are in your salad making, the more likely you are to have a highly nutritious meal. For example, don't stick to iceberg lettuce as your salad base. Dark green vegetables such as fresh spinach, romaine lettuce, endive, parsley, and red lettuce are more nutritious than iceberg lettuce and make a beautiful presentation.

You can make salads from a variety of raw vegetables. Use turnips, beets, green beans, radishes, carrots, cauliflower, avocados, red peppers, water chestnuts, zucchini, snow peas, and jicama. Garnish with sprouts, soy bits, seeds, croutons, and nuts. Cooked beans such as kidney, pinto, and garbanzo are great sources of protein that can be added to your salad. A small amount of shrimp or fish can be added for a more filling salad.

Avoid store-bought salad dressings. Many contain MSG, sugar, and undesirable chemicals and oils. Many women find that these additives worsen their anxiety symptoms. You can make your own dressings with cold-pressed oils, lemon juice, or vinegar. Add the dressing just before serving or serve it on the side so that diners can choose their own. Avoid the thick, creamy dressings that are high in calories and fat.

Sandwiches

Especially for lunches, many women prefer to buy premade sandwiches at a grocery store or deli or to make their own for a quick, easy-to-fix meal. Unfortunately, if not planned carefully, the fillings can be laden with high-salt and high-fat ingredients such as cheese, cream cheese, sausage, hot dogs, bologna, and salami, or rich dressings such as Thousand Island. Fats are difficult to digest, are dangerous for your cardiovascular system, and can cause excess weight gain. For a healthy sandwich the filling should contain a variety of nutritious vegetables such as lettuce, tomatoes, onion, sprouts, and avocados, used either as garnishes or as the sandwich base. Lean meats such as turkey, chicken (without the skin), and water-packed tuna are high in protein and low in calories. Also good are bean spreads such as soy, hummus (made from garbanzo beans), and tahini (made from sesame seeds). If sandwiches are your preferred type of quick meal, be sure to avoid rich, buttery breads such as croissants and brioches. The average croissant, for example, is over 50 percent butterfat.

Vegetables

Vegetables are important accompaniments to main courses like grains, beans, meat, and fish, and can help balance your meals properly. When prepared by themselves (not in a soup or salad), vegetables should be eaten raw or lightly steamed for optimal nutrition. Don't boil, cook in heavy oil, or cover vegetables with sauce. The high nutrient value of the vegetables is either lost or compromised with high-stress ingredients. Excellent vegetables for women suffering from anxiety and stress are listed in the following paragraphs.

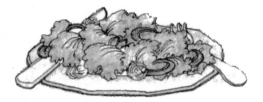

Leafy green vegetables. Kale, spinach, collards, turnip greens, mustard greens, and beet greens are packed with nutrients such as calcium, magnesium, and iron. Lightly steam (never boil) greens until tender but not soggy. After steaming, dress them with a mixture of olive oil, lemon juice, and a touch of sea salt. Other options include dressing greens with vinegar or a low-salt soy sauce.

Broccoli, cabbage, brussels sprouts, and cauliflower. These vegetables are good sources of minerals and are also excellent sources of nutrients like vitamin C that help the body to cope better with stress. They also contain chemicals that may protect the body from serious illnesses like cancer. They are delicious steamed and lightly dressed with lemon juice or with a combination of flax oil and a low-salt soy sauce. Broccoli can also be eaten raw or used in salads.

Root vegetables. Rutabagas, turnips, parsnips, beets, and sweet potatoes are packed with important vitamins and minerals. Many root vegetables are also used in other cultures and in macrobiotic healing models as sources of concentrated nutrients and as stabilizing and "grounding" foods. Root vegetables can be steamed or baked and served whole, mashed, or julienned (cut into long strips like french fries). Many women eat these vegetables rarely or only on holidays. I would recommend enjoying them much more often.

Squash. This delicious vegetable is easy to digest and low in calories. Many types of squash tend to be good sources of vitamins A and C. They are excellent sources of potassium. They are an ideal low-stress food for women combating anxiety, and you can use them in many different dishes. Baking squash makes it dry and stringy. Here are two better ways to prepare it:

> Steam until soft, then puree the squash in a blender. The resulting puree will be soft, smooth, and a beautiful golden color. The pureeing breaks down the complex carbohydrates so that it is surprisingly sweet and delicious—the taste is similar to sweet potatoes. You may want to add nutmeg and cinnamon for flavor.

> Slice the squash and sauté in olive oil, soy sauce, or broth.

Carrots and celery. These are members of the same food family. Both are delicious eaten raw, especially if kept crisp and chilled. They are also tasty when sliced and steamed. Eat carrots with a small amount of maple syrup to enhance their sweetness. Celery is delicious with onions or parsley.

Grains, Starches, and Legumes

Served together, grains, starches, and legumes are a chief source of complex carbohydrates and proteins for your lunch and dinner. Grains and beans are filling and slow to digest, and they tend to stabilize the blood sugar level; all are excellent foods for women in menopause and women with blood sugar imbalances or PMS-related anxiety symptoms. Because the long preparation time may discourage you from cooking beans and grains, here is a method to speed up the cooking time for beans:

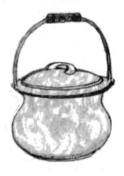

> Bring water to a boil (3 cups of water for every cup of beans). Add the beans to the boiling water and cook for two minutes. Remove from heat, partially cover pan, let beans stand for one hour. Go about your business or chores during this time as the beans are cooking themselves. After one hour, drain and rinse with cold water and then freeze. When you are ready to use the beans for a

meal, thaw them quickly under running water or in the microwave. In a large pot, boil 5 cups of water for every cup of beans. Add the beans to the boiling water. Lower the heat and cook covered for 30 to 50 minutes. The beans will then be ready.

Many types of beans, with low or no added salt, are available in cans. Health food stores also offer several brands of canned beans grown without pesticides or herbicides, a real plus for women who are very chemically sensitive.

Brown rice and other grains. You can prepare these grains in large quantities, then store them for several days in the refrigerator in a jar or plastic container. Reheat and use as needed. To reheat rice, place it over a double boiler or in a steamer, and cook for three to five minutes.

Potatoes. Potatoes are extremely easy to digest if baked or steamed. The problem with potatoes is the garnishes many people use, such as butter, sour cream, and bacon. Instead, use chives, sunflower seeds, and other no-salt seasonings. In place of butter try flax oil. It is delicious and you can use as much as you wish to make a fabulous baked potato. Potatoes can also be stuffed with leftover vegetables, with broth added for extra flavor.

Meat and Fish

Fish is an ideal food for women with anxiety and stress because of its high essential fatty acid content, which helps to decrease emotional stress and muscle tension. This is because the fatty acids contained in fish (particularly trout, salmon, tuna, and mackerel) are used by the body to produce the relaxant prostaglandin hormones found in tissues throughout the body. Fish are also good sources of stress-relieving minerals.

If you feel the need to eat meat other than fish, poultry is preferable. Serve boiled or roasted and without the skin. Avoid heavy sauces or dressings. Fish and poultry should be eaten more frequently than beef, pork, or lamb, which are higher in fat content. American dinners traditionally have been organized around a large piece of meat or fish, which formed the focal point, with small servings of grain and vegetables as side dishes. Women who want to enjoy optimal health throughout their lifetimes, should reverse the ratio. Keep your meat portions small (3 oz.) and fill up with a variety of other nutritious side dishes and always get lean cuts and trim off all visible fat. Most people eat much more meat protein than necessary. In large quantities, meat is hard to digest and can increase fatigue in many women.

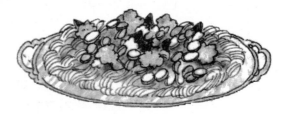

Combination Plates

One-dish meals can be a great choice for women with anxiety and stress. In these dishes a variety of foods are combined for both ease of preparation and taste. Vegetables and grains are the main ingredients, with meat used more as a flavoring (cut into small pieces and added to soups, salads, casseroles, and stir-fried dishes). Examples of such combinations would include chicken soup with rice and vegetables, tacos with beans, shredded chicken or shrimp on a corn tortilla. The taco provides three good sources of high-quality protein: meat, beans, and grain; and it is more nutritious served with added vegetables and sauce.

Casseroles should not be made with cheese (except nondairy cheese such as soy cheese) or butter-based sauces, but with more nutritious sauces. For example, puree vegetables such as broccoli, cauliflower, or carrots, and then blend the puree with chicken broth for a creamy sauce. Add arrowroot powder, rice flour, or buckwheat flakes as a thickener. Tofu may also be blended into the sauce for extra creaminess.

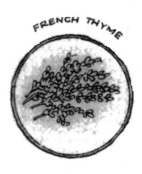

FRENCH THYME

Spices

Avoid black pepper, table salt, sugar, and monosodium glutamate (MSG), which are highly stressful to the body and can increase anxiety. Instead, use the milder herbs such as basil, thyme, dill, and tarragon. If you must use the stronger spices, use only one-fourth to one-half the amount called for in the recipe.

Lunch and Dinner Menus

These menus give you a variety of ways to organize your meals. Use them as guidelines as you create your own menus. The recipes for dishes marked with an asterisk are provided at the end of this chapter.

Soup Meals

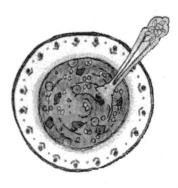

1   Vegetable soup*
    Rye bread
    Sliced tomatoes

2   Tomato soup
    Steamed potato
    Green beans
    Pear

3   Lentil soup*
    Brown rice
    Broccoli with lemon
    Romaine salad
    Banana

4   Miso soup
    Brown rice
    Lettuce salad

5   Split pea soup*
    Corn bread
    Green salad
    Applesauce

6   Onion soup
    Rye bread
    Romaine salad
    Lemon ice

Salad Meals

1 Mixed vegetable salad with
      kidney beans and
      sunflower seeds
   Whole grain bread

2 Apple and walnut salad
   Celery sticks
   Rye muffins

3 Guacamole with fresh
      vegetables
   Corn chips (unsalted)
   Fresh fruit combination

4 Potato salad
   Mixed bean salad
   Watermelon

5 Garbanzo bean and
      pasta salad with
      vinaigrette dressing
   Whole grain bread

6 Rice tabouli*
   Cucumber slices

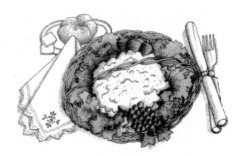

Sandwich Meals

1 Almond butter and jam
   Whole grain bread
   Sliced bananas

2 Tuna salad sandwich
   Rye bread
   Coleslaw

3 Avocado and romaine
      lettuce sandwich
   Oatmeal cookies

4 Hummus and tahini*
   Pita bread
   Tomato and
      cucumber slices

5 Soy cheese, lettuce,
      and tomato sandwich
   Rice bread
   Celery and carrot sticks

6 Vegeburger
   Whole green beans
   Lettuce, onions, tomato slices

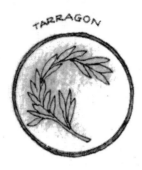
TARRAGON

Meat Meals

1 Broiled trout
  Steamed green beans
  Baked russet potato
  Mixed green salad

2 Poached salmon*
  Broccoli with lemon
  Steamed carrots
  Sliced tomatoes

3 Grilled shrimp
  Brown rice
  Snow peas
  Sliced tomatoes and cucumbers

4 Poached halibut
  Steamed red potatoes
  Crookneck squash
  Peas

5 Broiled tuna*
  Brown rice
  Romaine lettuce salad

6 Grilled sole
  Millet
  Zucchini squash
  Cole slaw

One-Dish Meals

1 Tofu, red peppers, onions,
    and celery stir-fry with rice
  Low-salt soy sauce

2 Vegetarian tacos, with bean,
    red pepper, avocado, onion,
    lettuce, and tomato filling*
  Low-salt salsa

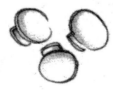

3 Pasta with mixed vegetables and
    tomato sauce

*The recipes for starred items are in the
next section of this chapter.*

4 Buckwheat with pinto
    beans, zucchini squash,
    and onions
  Low-salt tomato sauce

5 Shrimp, snow peas, and
    almond stir-fry with rice
  Low-salt soy sauce

6 Pasta with olive oil, garlic,
    and pine nuts
  Side vegetables
    (broccoli, green beans)

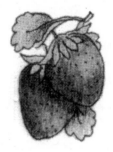

Healthy Breakfast Options

- Beverages
- Fruit
- Grains—cereals, muffins, and bread
- Spreads
- Raw nuts and seeds

Healthy Lunch and Dinner Options

- Beverages—mineral water, herbal tea, juice, roasted grain beverage, near-beer (nonalcoholized)
- Soup
- Salad and dressing
- Sandwich
- Grains and starches
- Vegetables
- Fish, poultry (small amounts)
- One-dish meals
- Low-stress dessert

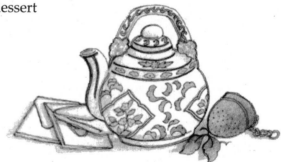

Recipes

Relaxant Tea   *Serves 2*

1 pint water
1 teaspoon
   chamomile leaves
1 teaspoon
   peppermint leaves
1 teaspoon honey
   (if desired)

Bring the water to boil. Place herbs in water and stir. Turn heat to low and steep for 15 minutes. Peppermint and chamomile help to relax and calm the mood. They are both muscle relaxants and antispasmodic herbs, so they can provide relief from anxiety-related muscle tension.

Flax Cereal with Bananas

Serves 1

6 tablespoons raw flax seeds
4–8 oz. nondairy vanilla milk
½ banana, sliced
sweetener (to taste)
cinnamon or nutmeg (to taste)

Grind raw flax seeds into a powder using a seed or coffee grinder. Place powder in a cereal bowl and slowly add the nondairy milk, stirring the mixture together. The flax mixture will thicken to a texture like cream of rice or oatmeal. Top the cereal with sliced bananas. Add sweetener if desired. Flax seeds are sensitive to light, air, and temperature, so eat this mixture right away. This cereal should be eaten cold; do not cook.

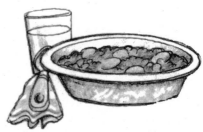

Nondairy Milk Breakfast Shake

Serves 2

2 cups nondairy milk
2 oz. soft tofu
3 tablespoons flax oil
1 large banana
¾ cup berries (strawberries, boysenberries, blueberries, or raspberries)

Combine all ingredients in a blender. Blend until smooth and serve. This delicious, creamy shake is excellent for relief from anxiety-related muscle tension and helps to calm the mood because it is high in essential fatty acids, calcium, vitamin C, and potassium.

High-Protein Flax Shake

Serves 2

6 tablespoons raw flax seeds
2 bananas
6 oz. water
6 oz. apple juice
1 tablespoon of vegetarian (soy- or rice-based) protein powder

Grind flax seeds to a powder using a coffee or seed grinder. Place the powdered flax seeds in a blender. Add the remaining ingredients and blend. Because of the whole flax seed, this recipe is high in essential fatty acids, calcium, magnesium, and potassium, which help relieve nervous tension.

Tofu Muesli Cereal
Serves 2

4 oz. soft tofu
2 oz. nondairy vanilla milk
2 tablespoons flax oil
1 banana
1 apple
15 raw almonds
sweetener (if desired)

Combine all ingredients in a food processor. Blend until creamy. Pour into a bowl and serve. This is a helpful cereal for nervous tension, high in essential fatty acids, calcium, magnesium, and potassium.

Vegetable Soup
Serves 6

4 tomatoes, diced
1 onion, chopped
1 turnip, chopped
1/2 leek, chopped
1 cup green peas
2 carrots, chopped
8 mushrooms, sliced
1 bay leaf
1/2 tablespoon thyme
1/2 tablespoon oregano
1 to 1-1/2 quarts water
1/4 bunch parsley, chopped
1/2 teaspoon salt substitute

Place all ingredients in a pot. Cover with the water. Bring to a boil, then turn heat to low. Cook for 2 hours. Pour the soup into individual serving dishes. Garnish with chopped parsley.

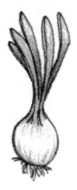

Lentil Soup
Serves 4

1 cup lentils
1/2 onion, chopped
1/2 cup carrots, chopped
1 to 1-1/2 quarts water
1 teaspoon brown rice miso

Wash lentils. Place all ingredients in a pot. Cover, bring to a boil, then turn heat to low and simmer until lentils are soft. Vary the amount of water depending on the desired thickness of the soup.

Split Pea Soup

Serves 4

1 cup split peas
½ onion, chopped
1 small carrot, sliced
1 quart water
¼ to ½ teaspoon sea salt
   or salt substitute

Wash peas. Place peas, onion, and carrot in a pot. Add the water. Cover, bring to a boil, then turn heat to low. Cook for 45 minutes. Add sea salt and continue to cook until peas are soft. Soup may be cooled and then pureed in a blender if you prefer a creamy texture.

Rice Tabouli

Serves 6

2 cups cooked brown rice
1 cup parsley, chopped
½ cup fresh mint, chopped
½ medium red onion, diced
1 medium tomato, diced
juice of 1 lemon
2 tablespoons olive oil
1 teaspoon cumin
1 teaspoon oregano
¼ teaspoon salt

Place rice in a bowl. Mix in parsley, mint, red onion, and tomato. Combine well. Add lemon juice and olive oil and mix. Add cumin, oregano, and salt to the salad; mix well. This is a delicious and healthy tabouli recipe.

Hummus and Tahini

Serves 4

¾ cup raw unhulled
   sesame seeds
1 cup water or cooking
   liquid from beans
1-¾ cup garbanzo beans,
   cooked
juice of 1 lemon
2 tablespoons olive oil
1 clove of raw garlic
¼ teaspoon salt

Grind sesame seeds into a powder using a seed or coffee grinder. (Raw sesame butter, which is available from most health food stores, may be substituted.) Combine water, garbanzo beans, ground sesame seeds, lemon juice, olive oil, garlic, and salt in a food processor. Blend until it is the consistency of a smooth dip. Use as a sandwich filling with lettuce and tomatoes in pita bread. You can serve it as a dip with pita bread, rye bread, and fresh vegetables.

Poached Salmon

Serves 4

1 cup water
1 lemon
4 fillets of salmon, 3 oz. each

Combine water and juice of one lemon in skillet and heat. Place the salmon in the hot liquid. Cover and poach for 6 to 8 minutes or until the salmon flakes easily with a fork. Remove the fish and keep it warm until you are ready to serve.

Broiled Tuna

Serves 4

4 fillets of tuna, 4 oz. each
1 tablespoon canola oil
2 tablespoons lemon juice

Baste the tuna fillets with oil and then sprinkle with lemon juice. Place the tuna in a broiler pan. Broil for 5 to 6 minutes, or until done to your satisfaction.

Vegetarian Tacos

Serves 4

4 corn tortillas
¾ pound pinto beans, cooked
    and pureed
½ avocado, thinly sliced
¼ sweet red pepper, diced
1 tomato, diced
¼ red onion, finely chopped
½ head red or romaine lettuce,
    chopped
6 tablespoons salsa

Warm tortillas and beans in separate pans. Place tortillas on individual serving dishes and spread with beans. Garnish with avocado, pepper, tomato, and onion, then cover each taco with lettuce and 1-½ tablespoons of salsa.

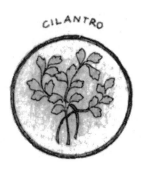

CILANTRO

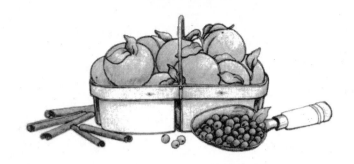

Substitute Healthy Ingredients in Recipes

Learning how to make substitutions for high-stress ingredients in familiar recipes allows you to prepare your favorite foods without compromising your emotional or physical health. Many recipes contain ingredients that women with anxiety and stress should avoid, particularly the high-stress foods such as caffeine, alcohol, sugar, chocolate, and dairy products. By replacing these with healthier ingredients, you can continue to make many recipes that appeal to you. I have recommended this approach for years to my patients, who are pleased to find that they can still have their favorite dishes, but in much healthier versions.

Some women choose to totally eliminate high-stress ingredients from a recipe. For example, you can make a pasta with tomato sauce but eliminate the Parmesan cheese topping and use nonwheat pasta. Greek salad can be made without the feta cheese. Some of my patients even make pizza without cheese, layering tomato sauce and lots of vegetables on the crust. In many cases, the high-stress ingredients are not necessary to make foods taste good; always remember, they can worsen your anxiety symptoms and impair your health.

If you want to use a particular high-stress ingredient, you can usually substantially reduce the amount of that ingredient you use, while still retaining the flavor and taste. Most of us have palates jaded by too much fat, salt, sugar, and other flavorings. In many dishes, we taste only the additives; we never really enjoy the delicious flavors of the foods themselves. Now that I regularly substitute low-stress ingredients in my cooking, I enjoy the subtle taste of the dishes much more. Also, my health and vitality continue to improve with the deletion of high-stress ingredients. The following information tells you how to substitute healthy ingredients in your own recipes. The substitutions are simple to make and should benefit your health greatly.

Substitutions for Caffeinated Foods and Beverages

Drink substitutes for coffee and black tea.
The best substitutes are the grain-based coffee beverages, such as Pero™, Postum™, and Cafix™. Some women may find the abrupt discontinuance of coffee too difficult because of withdrawal symptoms, such as headaches. If this concerns you, decrease your total coffee intake gradually to only one or one-half cup per day and use grain-based substitutes for your other cups. This will help prevent withdrawal symptoms.

Drink decaffeinated coffee or tea during transition.
If you cannot give up coffee, start by substituting water-processed decaffeinated coffee for the real thing. Then try to wean yourself from coffee altogether, or go to a coffee substitute.

Use herbal teas for energy and vitality. Many women with anxiety and excessive stress mistakenly drink coffee as a pick-me-up to be able to function during the day. Use ginger instead. It is a great herbal stimulant that won't wreck your health. To make ginger tea, grate a few teaspoons of fresh ginger root into a pot of hot water; boil and steep. Serve with honey.

Substitute carob for chocolate. Unsweetened carob tastes like chocolate but doesn't contain the anxiety-worsening caffeine found in chocolate. A member of the legume family, carob is high in calcium. You can purchase it in chunk form as a substitute for chocolate candy or as a powder for use in baking or drinks. Be careful, however, not to overindulge; carob, like chocolate, is high in calories and fat. Consider it a treat and a cooking aid for use in small amounts only.

Substitutions for Sugar

Substitute concentrated sweeteners. Americans tend to be addicted to sugar, which can worsen anxiety symptoms. Most of us grew up on highly sugared soft drinks, candy, and rich pastries—no wonder the incidence of diabetes is soaring among our population. I have found that as women decrease their sugar intake, most begin to really enjoy the subtle flavors of the foods they eat. Concentrated sweeteners such as honey and maple syrup have a sweeter taste per quantity used than table sugar. Using these substitutes will allow you to decrease the amount of sweetener you use in a recipe. If you use a concentrated sweetener in place of sugar in an ordinary recipe, reduce the liquid content in the recipe by one-fourth cup. If no liquid is used in the recipe, add 3 to 5 tablespoons of flour for each three-fourths cup of concentrated sweetener.

Substitute fruit for sugar in pastries. In making muffins and cookies, you may want to try deleting sugar altogether and adding extra fruits and nuts.

Substitutions for Alcohol

Use low-alcohol or nonalcoholic products for drinking or cooking. There are many delicious low-alcohol and nonalcoholic wines and beers for sale in supermarkets and liquor stores. Many of these taste quite good and can be used for meals or at social occasions. In addition, you can substitute low-alcohol or nonalcoholic wine or beer when cooking or preparing sauces and marinades. You will retain much of the flavor that alcohol imparts, and you'll decrease the stress factor substantially.

Substitutions for Dairy Products

Eliminate or decrease the amount of cow's milk cheese you use in food preparation and cooking. If you must use cow's milk cheese in cooking, decrease the amount in the recipe by three-fourths so that it becomes a flavoring or garnish rather than a major source of fat and protein. For example, use one teaspoon of Parmesan cheese on top of a casserole instead of one-half cup.

Use soy cheese in food preparation and cooking. Soy cheese is an excellent substitute for cow's milk cheese. It is lower in fat and salt, and the fat it does contain isn't saturated. Health food stores offer many brands that come in many different flavors, such as mozzarella, cheddar, American, and jack. The quality of these products keeps improving all the time. You can use soy cheese as a perfect cheese substitute in sandwiches, salads, pizzas, lasagnas, and casseroles. In some recipes you can replace cheese with soft tofu. I have done this often with lasagna, layering the lasagna noodles with tofu and topping with melted soy cheese for a delicious dish. The tofu, which is bland, takes on the taste of the tomato sauce.

Replace milk and yogurt in recipes. For cow's milk, substitute potato milk, soy milk, nut milk, or grain milk. One of my personal favorites is a nondairy milk called Vance's Darifree that is made from an all-vegetable potato base. It is easily digestible and particularly good for women with anxiety and other symptoms as well as fatigue. It is creamy and sweet and tastes very similar to the best cow's milk, with none of the unhealthy characteristics of dairy products. Even my twelve-year-old daughter likes it. The potato-based milk is high in calcium and can be purchased dry or homogenized in the dairy section of your local supermarket. It mixes easily in water and can be used exactly as you use cow's milk for beverages, cooking, and baking. Soy milk is particularly good and comes in many flavors. Many nondairy milks are good sources of calcium and can be used for drinking, eating, or baking. Potato, soy and nut milks are available at most health food stores.

For cow's milk–based yogurt, substitute soy yogurt. Several excellent brands of soy yogurt are available in health food stores in plain, vanilla, and fruit flavors. The taste is excellent and approximates that of cow's milk yogurt. Soy yogurt is a good substitute for both cooking and baking.

Substitute flax oil for butter. Flax oil is the best substitute for butter I've found; it's a rich, golden oil that looks and tastes quite a bit like butter. It is delicious on anything you'd normally top with butter—toast, rice, popcorn, steamed vegetables, or potatoes. Flax oil is extremely high in essential fatty acids—the type of fat that is very healthy for a woman's body. Essential fatty acids improve vitality, enhance circulation, and help promote normal hormonal function. Flax oil is quite perishable, however, because it is sensitive to heat and light. You can't cook with it—cook the food first and add the flax oil before serving. Also, keep it refrigerated. Flax oil has so many health benefits that I highly recommend its use. You can find it in health food stores.

Substitutions for Red Meat and Poultry

Substitute beans, tofu, or seeds in recipes. You can often modify recipes calling for hamburger or ground turkey by substituting tofu. For example, crumble up the tofu to simulate the texture of hamburger and add to recipes for enchiladas, tacos, chili, and ground beef casseroles. The tofu takes on the flavor of the sauce used in the dish and is indistinguishable from meat. I do this often when cooking at home. In addition, many substitute meat products are available in natural food stores. These products include tofu hot dogs, hamburgers, bacon, ham, chicken, and turkey. The variety is astounding, and many of these fake meat products taste remarkably good. The quality of these products has dramatically improved.

When making salads that call for meat, such as chef's salad or Cobb salad, substitute kidney beans and garbanzo beans, along with sunflower seeds. These will provide the needed protein, yet be more easily digestible. You can also sprinkle sunflower seeds on top of casseroles for extra protein and essential fatty acids. When making stir-fries, substitute tofu, almonds, or sprouts for beef or chicken. Vegetable protein-based stir-fries taste delicious!

Substitutions for Wheat Flour

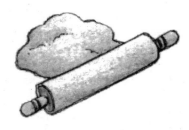

Use whole grain, nonwheat flour.   Substitute whole grain, non-wheat flours, such as rice or barley flour. Whole grain flours are much higher than refined flours in essential nutrients, such as the vitamin B complex and many minerals. They are also higher in fiber content. Rice flour makes excellent cookies, cakes, and other pastries. Barley flour is best used for pie crusts.

Substitutions for Salt

Substitute potassium-based products for table salt (sodium chloride).   Potassium-based products, such as Morton's Salt Substitute™, are much healthier and will not aggravate heart disease or hypertension.

Use powdered seaweeds such as kelp or nori to season vegetables, grains, and salads.   They are high in essential iodine and trace elements.

Use herbs instead of salt for flavoring.   Their flavors are much more subtle and will help even the most jaded palate appreciate the taste of fresh fruits, vegetables, and meats.

Use liquid flavoring agents with advertised low-sodium content.   Low-salt soy sauce and Bragg's Amino Acids™, a liquid soybean-based flavoring agent, are delicious when used as salt substitutes in cooking. Add them to soups, casseroles, stir-fries, and other dishes at the end of the cooking process. You need only a small amount for intense flavoring.

Substitutes for Common High-Stress Ingredients

High-Stress Ingredient	Low-Stress Substitute
¾ cup sugar	½ cup honey
	¼ cup molasses
	½ cup maple syrup
	½ oz. barley malt
	1 cup apple butter
	2 cups apple juice
1 cup milk	1 cup soy, potato, nut, or grain milk
1 cup yogurt	1 cup soy yogurt
1 tablespoon butter	1 tablespoon flax oil (must be used raw and unheated)
½ teaspoon salt	1 tablespoon miso
	½ teaspoon potassium chloride salt substitute
	½ teaspoon Mrs. Dash™, Spike™
	½ teaspoon herbs (basil, tarragon, oregano, etc.)
1-½ cups cocoa	1 cup powdered carob
1 square chocolate	¾ tablespoon powdered carob
1 tablespoon coffee	1 tablespoon decaffeinated coffee
	1 tablespoon Pero™, Postum™, Caffix™, or other grain-based coffee substitute
4 oz. wine	4 oz. light wine
8 oz. beer	8 oz. near beer
1 cup wheat flour	1 cup barley flour (pie crust)
	1 cup rice flour (cookies, cakes, breads)
1 cup meat	1 cup beans, tofu
	¼ cup seeds

5

Vitamins, Minerals, Herbs & Essential Fatty Acids

Nutritional supplements can play an important role in your anxiety and stress recovery program. They can help stabilize and relax your mood, promoting a sense of peace and calm. In addition, they can help promote optimal function of your immune system, glands, and digestive tract. They can also stimulate good circulation of blood and oxygen to the entire body, a necessity for high energy and vitality. When adequate nutritional support is lacking, I have found it very difficult to relieve anxiety symptoms entirely. Because poor or inadequate nutrition may play a major role in causing anxiety, essential nutrients are an important facet of a good program for anxiety and stress treatment. Numerous research studies done at university centers and hospitals support the importance of nutrition in relieving stress; a bibliography is included at the end of this chapter for those wanting more technical information.

Most women have difficulty increasing their nutrient intake up to the levels needed for optimal healing using diet alone. Supplements can help make up this deficiency so you feel better as rapidly and completely as possible. I do want to emphasize the importance of a good diet along with the use of supplements. Supplements should never be used as an excuse to continue poor dietary habits. I have found that my patients heal most effectively when they combine a nutrient-rich diet with the right mix of supplements.

This chapter is divided into four sections. The first discusses the role of vitamins and minerals in decreasing anxiety and stress symptoms; the second section tells which herbs help relieve anxiety. The third section explains the benefits of essential fatty acids. I end the chapter with specific recommendations on how to make and use your own supplements, along with a series of charts that list major food sources for each essential nutrient.

Vitamins and Minerals for Relief of Anxiety

Many vitamins and minerals are useful in the treatment and prevention of anxiety. This section contains complete information on those supplements that provide the most symptom relief.

Vitamin B Complex.   This complex consists of 11 separate B vitamins that are often found together in food. In many cases they participate in the same chemical reactions in the body; therefore, they need to be taken together for the best results. The B vitamins play an important role in healthy nervous system function. When one or more of these vitamins are deficient, symptoms of nerve impairment as well as anxiety, stress, and fatigue can result. Conversely, adequate intake of these nutrients can help to calm the mood and provide important components of a stable and constant source of energy.

B-complex vitamins also help regulate the mood and emotional well-being, by facilitating carbohydrate metabolism and the cellular conversion of glucose to usable energy (ATP). Certain B vitamins help promote cell respiration, so the cells can use oxygen efficiently. In addition, B vitamins are needed for healthy liver function. When they are deficient, the liver is unable to efficiently perform its role as the body's chief detoxifying organ. This role includes the inactivation of estrogen. When excessive levels of estrogen accumulate in the body, it acts as a brain stimulant, worsening symptoms of anxiety and nervous tension. B vitamins are also necessary to enable the liver to detoxify alcohol. Excessive alcohol consumption can deplete vitamin B_{12} and folic acid as well as other vitamins in the B family.

Deficiencies of individual B vitamins also increase anxiety and stress. Pantothenic acid (vitamin B_5) is needed for healthy adrenal function. High emotional stress triggers the fight-or-flight alarm response in the body, which includes excessive output of adrenal hormones. Pyridoxine (vitamin B_6) also affects moods through its important role in the conversion of linoleic acid to gamma linolenic acid (GLA) in the production of the beneficial series-one prostaglandins. Prostaglandins have a relaxant effect on both mood and smooth muscle tissue. Lack of these relaxant hormones has been linked to PMS-related anxiety, menstrual cramps, and stress-related problems like irritable bowel syndrome and migraine headaches.

Using the birth control pill, a common treatment for PMS, menstrual cramps, and irregularity, decreases vitamin B_6 levels. Menopausal women on estrogen replacement therapy are also at risk of B_6 deficiency. Anxiety symptoms can occur as a side effect of hormone use in both groups of women, in part because of B_6 deficiency. B_6 supplementation may help reduce these symptoms. B_6 can be safely used in doses up to 300 mg. Doses above this level can be neurotoxic and should be avoided.

Lack of B_6 may also increase anxiety symptoms directly through its effect on the nervous system. B_6 is needed for the conversion of the amino acid tryptophan to serotonin, an important neurotransmitter. Serotonin regulates sleep, and when it is deficient, insomnia occurs. Sleeplessness is a condition often seen in anxious women. Serotonin levels also strongly affect mood and social behavior. Both B_6 and food sources of tryptophan such as almonds, pumpkin seeds, sesame seeds, and certain other protein-containing foods are necessary for adequate serotonin production.

For those women who fall asleep easily but can't return to sleep after awakening in the middle of the night, niacin (vitamin B_3) may be helpful. Research studies have shown that niacinamide, a form of niacin, has effects similar to those of the minor tranquilizers. In addition, inositol, another B vitamin, has been shown to have calming effects. Its effect on the brain waves studied by electroencephalograph (EEG) was also similar to changes induced by minor tranquilizers.

In summary, the entire range of B vitamins is needed to provide nutritional support for anxiety and stress symptoms. Because B vitamins are water soluble, the body cannot readily store them. Thus, B vitamins must be taken in daily in the diet. Women who are anxious and experiencing significant stress should eat foods high in B vitamins and use vitamin supplements. Good sources of most B vitamins include brewer's yeast (which many women cannot digest readily), liver, whole grain germ and bran, beans, peas, and nuts. B_{12} is found mainly in animal foods. Women following a vegan diet (a vegetarian diet utilizing no dairy products or eggs) should take particular care to add supplemental vitamin B_{12} to their diets.

Vitamin C. This is an extremely important antistress nutrient that can help decrease the fatigue symptoms that often accompany excessive levels of anxiety and stress. It is needed for the production of adrenal gland hormones. When the fight-or-flight pattern is activated in response to stress, these hormones become depleted. Larger amounts of vitamin C in the diet are needed when stress levels are high. In one research study done on 411 dentists and their spouses, scientists found a clear relationship between lack of vitamin C and the presence of fatigue.

By supporting the immune function, vitamin C helps prevent fatigue caused by infections. It stimulates the production of interferon, a chemical that prevents the spread of viruses in the body. Necessary for healthy white blood cells and their antibody production, vitamin C also helps the body fight bacterial and fungal infections. Women with low vitamin C intake tend to have elevated levels of histamine, a chemical that triggers allergy symptoms. Allergy attacks can be the cause of emotional symptoms like anxiety.

Vitamin C has also been tested, along with bioflavonoids, as a treatment for anemia caused by heavy menstrual bleeding—a common cause of fatigue and depression in teenagers and pre-menopausal women in their forties. Vitamin C reduces bleeding by helping to strengthen capillaries and prevent capillary fragility. One clinical study of vitamin C showed a reduction in bleeding in 87 percent of women taking supplemental amounts of this essential nutrient. By strengthening the capillaries, vitamin C improves the metabolism of all the systems in the body. Healthy blood vessels permit better flow of nutrients into the cells, as well as facilitating the flow of waste products out of the cells. This is necessary for optimal health and well-being.

The best sources of vitamin C in nature are fruits and vegetables. It is a water-soluble vitamin, so it is not stored in the body. Thus, women with anxiety and excessive stress should replenish their vitamin C supply daily through a healthy diet and the use of supplements.

Bioflavonoids. In nature, bioflavonoids often occur with vitamin C in fruits and vegetables. For example, they are found in grape skins, cherries, blackberries, and blueberries. Bioflavonoids are abundant in citrus fruits, especially in the pulp and the white rind. They are also found in other foods such as buckwheat and soybeans. Along with vitamin C, bioflavonoids strengthen the cells of small blood vessels and prevent anemia due to heavy menstrual bleeding, a common cause of fatigue and depression.

Bioflavonoids have the additional property of being weakly estrogenic and antiestrogenic, important properties for control of anxiety and stress due to hormonal deficiency (menopause) or hormonal imbalance (PMS). Bioflavonoids belong to a classification of estrogen-containing plants called "phytoestrogens." Other plants in this group include fennel, anise, and licorice. Though these plants are estrogenic, the doses found are much weaker than the levels in drugs. Though bioflavonoids contain 1/50,000 the potency of a drug dose of estrogen, such plant sources of estrogen can compete with the estrogen precursors produced by your body for space on the binding sites of enzymes needed for estrogen production. Thus, on one hand, bioflavonoids can lower excessive estrogen levels that trigger PMS and other health problems such as fibroids and endometriosis. On the other hand, the weakly estrogenic effect of the bioflavonoids can actually help relieve symptoms such as hot flashes, night sweats, anxiety, mood swings, and insomnia in menopausal women grossly deficient in estrogen. One study researching the beneficial effects of bioflavonoids on menopausal women was done in Chicago during the 1960s at Loyola University Medical School. The study showed that bioflavonoids were very effective in decreasing hot flashes. In summary, the bioflavonoids actually help to normalize estrogen levels in a variety of gynecological conditions. This can help decrease symptoms of anxiety and stress that are linked to hormonal imbalances.

Vitamin E.　Like bioflavonoids, vitamin E relieves symptoms of anxiety and mood swings triggered by an estrogen-progesterone imbalance. This can occur in women suffering from either PMS or menopause. In studies of vitamin E as an alternative treatment for menopause, it has relieved hot flashes, night sweats, mood swings, and even vaginal dryness. Women who find that conventional estrogen therapy actually worsens their anxiety symptoms (because the available drug doses do not match their body's needs) are also potentially good candidates for vitamin E therapy. In women suffering from PMS, vitamin E helped alleviate anxiety, mood swings, and food craving symptoms. In several controlled studies, it has also been found to help reduce fibrocystic breast lumps and breast tenderness.

Vitamin E is a very important nutrient for women's health. The best natural sources of vitamin E are wheat germ oil, walnut oil, soy bean oil, and other grain and seed oils. I generally recommend that women with menopause and PMS-related anxiety use between 400 to 2000 I.U. per day. Women with hypertension, diabetes, or bleeding problems should start on a much lower dose of vitamin E (100 I.U. per day). If you have any of these conditions, ask your physician about the advisability of using these supplements. Any increase in dosage should be made slowly and monitored carefully in these women. Otherwise, vitamin E tends to be extremely safe and is commonly used by millions of people.

Magnesium. The body requires adequate levels of magnesium in order to maintain energy and vitality. Women suffering from excessive levels of anxiety experience increased levels of stress and wear and tear on the body and depleted energy levels. The body needs magnesium in order to produce ATP, the end product of the conversion of food to usable energy by the body's cells. ATP is the universal energy currency that the body uses to run hundreds of thousands of chemical reactions. The digestive system can efficiently extract this energy from food only in the presence of magnesium, oxygen, and other nutrients. When magnesium is deficient, ATP production falls and the body forms lactic acid instead. Researchers have linked excessive accumulation of lactic acid with anxiety and irritability symptoms.

Magnesium is also needed to facilitate both the conversion of the essential fatty acid linoleic acid to gamma linolenic acid and the conversion of gamma linolenic acid to the beneficial relaxant prostaglandin hormones. Stimulating production of these hormones helps to reduce the anxiety and mood swing symptoms of PMS, eating disorders, and agoraphobia (fear of public places). Research has found magnesium deficiencies in the red blood cells of women suffering from PMS. In one study of 192 women, magnesium nitrate was given one week premenstrually and during the first two days of menstruation. Nervous tension was relieved in 89 percent of the women studied. These women also noted relief of headaches, breast tenderness, and weight gain. Interestingly enough, deficiency of magnesium has also been found to cause signs of stress in the adrenal gland. This is noteworthy since the adrenal gland helps to mediate physiological stress in the body.

Medical research studies in the treatment of chronic fatigue use a special form of magnesium called magnesium aspartate, formed by combining magnesium with aspartic acid. Aspartic acid also plays an important role in the production of energy in the body and helps transport magnesium and potassium into the cells. Magnesium aspartate, along with potassium aspartate, has been tested in a number of clinical studies and has been shown to reduce fatigue after five to six weeks of constant use. Many volunteers began to feel better even within ten days. This beneficial effect was seen in 90 percent of the people tested, a very high success rate.

Magnesium is an important nutrient for women with stress-related intestinal problems, particularly diarrhea and vomiting. A magnesium deficiency can develop if these symptoms are chronic. When a deficiency occurs, it can worsen anxiety, fatigue, weakness, confusion, and muscle tremor in susceptible women. Women with these symptoms must replace the magnesium through appropriate supplementation. Magnesium deficiency has also been seen in women suffering from PMS; medical studies have found a reduction in red blood cell magnesium during the second half of the menstrual cycle in affected women. Magnesium, like vitamin B_6, is needed for the production of the beneficial prostaglandin hormones as well as for glucose metabolism. Magnesium supplements can also benefit women with severe emotionally triggered anxiety and insomnia. When taken before bedtime, magnesium helps to calm the mood and induce restful sleep.

Good food sources of magnesium include green leafy vegetables, beans and peas, raw nuts and seeds, tofu, avocados, raisins, dried figs, and millet and other grains. For women who choose to use magnesium supplements, the optimal dose is 400 to 500 mg per day.

Potassium. Like magnesium, potassium has a powerful enhancing effect on energy and vitality. Potassium deficiency has been associated with fatigue and muscular weakness. One study showed that older people who were deficient in potassium had weaker grip strength. Potassium aspartate has been used with magnesium aspartate in a number of studies on chronic fatigue; this combination significantly restored energy levels.

Potassium has many important roles in the body. It constitutes 5 percent of the total mineral content of the body. It regulates the transfer of nutrients into the cells and works with sodium to maintain the body's water balance. Its role in water balance is important in preventing PMS bloating symptoms. Potassium aids proper muscle contraction and transmission of electrochemical impulses. It helps maintain nervous system function and a healthy heart rate. Potassium is commonly lost through chronic diarrhea or the excessive use of diuretics (which many women with PMS use to combat bloating around the time of their periods). In addition, the excessive use of coffee and alcohol (both of which can worsen anxiety and emotional stress symptoms) increases the loss of potassium through the urinary tract.

For women suffering from potassium loss, the use of a potassium supplement may be helpful. The most common dose available is a 99-mg tablet or capsule. I generally recommend one to three per day to be used up to one week premenstrually. Potassium, however, should be used cautiously. It should be avoided by women with kidney or cardiovascular disease, because a high level of potassium can cause an irregular heartbeat in women with these problems. Also, potassium can be irritating to the intestinal tract, so it should be taken with meals. If you have any questions about the proper use of this mineral, ask your health-care provider. Potassium occurs in abundance in fruits, vegetables, beans and peas, seeds and nuts, starches, and whole grains.

Calcium. Calcium is the most abundant mineral in the body. This important mineral helps combat stress, nervous tension, and anxiety. A calcium deficiency increases not only emotional irritability but also muscular irritability and cramps. Calcium can be taken at night along with magnesium to calm the mood and induce a restful sleep. This is particularly helpful for women with menopause-related anxiety, mood swings, and insomnia. Because calcium is a major structural component of bone, it has the added benefit of helping prevent bone loss, or osteoporosis.

Like magnesium and potassium, calcium is essential in the maintenance of regular heartbeat and the healthy transmission of impulses through the nerves. It may also help reduce blood pressure and regulate cholesterol levels; it is essential for blood clotting.

Many women do not take in the recommended daily allowance for calcium in their diet (800 mg for women during active reproductive years, 1200 mg after menopause). In fact, many women take in only half the recommended amount. Good sources of calcium include green leafy vegetables, salmon (with bones), nuts and seeds, tofu, and blackstrap molasses. In addition, a calcium supplement may be useful.

Zinc. This mineral helps decrease anxiety and stress by facilitating the action of B vitamins, creating proper blood sugar balance as well as healthy immune function, digestion, and metabolism. Zinc is an essential trace mineral necessary for the absorption and action of vitamins, especially the anxiety and stress-combating B vitamins. It is a constituent of many enzymes involved in metabolism and digestion. Zinc helps reduce the anxiety due to blood sugar imbalances since it plays a role in normal carbohydrate digestion. It is a component of insulin, the protein that helps move glucose out of the blood circulation and into the cells. Once inside the cells, glucose provides them with their main source of energy. In addition, zinc is part of the enzyme that is needed to break down alcohol. It is also necessary for the proper growth and development of the female reproductive tract and for effective wound healing. Zinc enhances the immune function, acting as an immune stimulant (it has been shown to trigger the reproduction of lymphocytes when incubated with these cells in a test tube). Finally, zinc is needed for the synthesis of nucleic acids, which control the production of the different proteins in the body. Good food sources of zinc include wheat germ, pumpkin seeds, whole grain products, wheat bran, and high-protein foods.

Chromium and Maganese. These two minerals are important in carbohydrate production and metabolism. Chromium helps keep the blood sugar level in balance by enhancing insulin function so glucose is properly utilized by the body. This prevents the extremes of too little glucose in the blood (hypoglycemia) or too much glucose (diabetes mellitus). By improving the intake of glucose into the cells, chromium helps the cells produce energy. Chromium accomplishes these functions through its participation in an important molecule called the glucose tolerance factor (GTF). GTF is composed of chromium, niacin (vitamin B3), and three amino acids—glycerin, cysteine, and glutamic acid. This combination allows chromium to be available in the body in a biologically active form. Good sources of chromium include brewer's yeast, whole wheat, rye, oysters, potatoes, apples, bananas, spinach, molasses, and chicken.

Manganese aids glucose metabolism by acting as a cofactor in the process of converting glucose (food) to energy. It is also important in the digestion of food, especially proteins, and in the production of cholesterol and fatty acids in the body. Manganese is also needed for healthy bone growth and development as well as the production of the thyroid hormone, thyroxin. Food sources of manganese include nuts and whole grains. Seeds, beans, peas, and leafy green vegetables are also good sources when they have been grown in soil containing manganese. Animal foods tend to be low in this essential nutrient.

Herbal Relief for Conditions Coexisting with Anxiety

Many herbs can help relieve the symptoms and treat the causes of anxiety and stress. I have used anxiety- and stress-relieving herbs in my practice for many years, and many women have found them to be effective remedies. I use them to extend the nutrition of a healthy diet. Herbs can balance and expand the diet while optimizing nutritional intake. Some herbs provide an additional source of nutrients that can relax tension and ease anxiety. Other herbs have mild immune-boosting and hormonal properties; they support the endocrine and the immune systems with a minimum of side effects. In this section, I describe many specific herbs useful for relief of anxiety and stress-related symptoms.

Herbs for Anxiety

Sedative and Relaxant Herbs.   Herbs such as valerian root, passionflower, hops, chamomile, and skullcap have a significant calming and restful effect on the central nervous system. Other calming herbs include bay, balm, catnip, celery, lavender, wild cherry, and yarrow; they all promote emotional calm and well-being. With their mild sedative effect, they also promote restful sleep, a state that is difficult to induce when a woman is suffering from excessive anxiety and stress. Passionflower has been found to elevate levels of the neurotransmitter serotonin. Serotonin is synthesized from tryptophan, an essential amino acid that has been shown in numerous medical studies to initiate restful sleep. Chamomile, an herb that makes delicate, tasty tea, is a good source of tryptophan. Valerian root has been used extensively in traditional herbal medicine as a sleep inducer and is widely used both in Europe and the United States as a gentle herbal remedy to help combat insomnia. Unfortunately, valerian has an unpleasant taste, making it more palatable when taken in capsule form.

I have been very pleased with the benefits these herbs have brought to my patients suffering from menopause-related anxiety and insomnia. Many women with moderate to severe symptoms of hormonal deficiency wake up two to three times a night. If you suffer from menopause-related insomnia, you may need to make a sedative tea like hops or chamomile fairly strong, using as many as two or three tea bags instead of one. Start with a weaker tea and increase the potency slowly until you find the level that works best for you.

Many women with anxiety also suffer from the unpleasant physical symptoms of tight, tense muscles in vulnerable areas of their bodies (neck, shoulders, jaw, and the upper and lower back are common areas to store tension). Many of these relaxant herbs help to relieve the muscle tension and spasm that often accompany stress. Certain herbs like valerian root, peppermint, and chamomile are also effective in relieving stress-related indigestion and intestinal gas.

Blood-Circulation Enhancers. Certain herbs such as ginger and ginkgo biloba improve circulation to the tight and tense muscles, thereby helping to relieve a common physiological response to anxiety. Ginger causes a widening or dilation of the blood vessels. Better blood circulation helps to draw nutrients to contracted, tense muscles and also helps to remove waste products like lactic acid and carbon dioxide. As muscle metabolism improves, tension symptoms diminish. Ginger also has an antispasmodic effect on the smooth muscle of the intestinal tract and can help relieve digestive symptoms of excessive levels of anxiety and stress.

Besides taking ginger in tincture or capsule form, you can drink it as a delicious tea. To make ginger tea, buy a fresh ginger root at your supermarket. Grate a few teaspoons of the fresh root into a quart pot of water. Boil and steep for 30 minutes. This is a very soothing herbal tea, delicious with a small amount of honey.

Ginkgo biloba also improves blood circulation and oxygenation to tense muscles. It has a vasodilating effect and decreases metabolic processes during a period of decreased blood supply. It is a very powerful herbal remedy and can be effectively combined with ginger.

Herbs for Chronic Fatigue and Depression

Many women with anxiety also suffer from depression and fatigue. Anxiety and panic episodes can be exhausting to the body, stressing the endocrine and immune systems, and other important systems. Many women feel tired and depleted after anxiety episodes, since these episodes use up the body's available energy and nutrients. Also, women suffering from PMS, menopause, and hypoglycemia and food allergies "roller coaster" between highs and lows, even during a single day.

A number of herbs can help a woman experiencing excessive fatigue due to anxiety episodes, PMS, and hypoglycemia. Herbs such as oat straw, ginger, ginkgo biloba, dandelion root, and Siberian ginseng (eleutherococcus) may have a stimulatory effect, improving energy and vitality. Women who use these herbs may note an increased ability to handle stress, as well as improved physical and mental capabilities.

Some of the salutary effects may be due to the high levels of essential nutrients captured in herbs. For example, dandelion root contains magnesium, potassium, and vitamin E, while ginkgo contains high levels of bioflavonoids. These essential nutrients help relieve fatigue, depression, PMS, and hot flashes, and they increase resistance to infections. Oat straw has been used to relieve fatigue and weakness, especially when there is an emotional component.

Siberian ginseng and ginger have been important traditional medicines in China and other countries for thousands of years. They have been reputed to increase longevity and decrease fatigue and weakness. In modern China, Japan, and other countries, there is a great deal of interest in the pharmacological effects of these traditional herbs. Scientific studies are corroborating the medicinal effects of these plants. These herbs boost immunity and strengthen the cardiovascular system. The bioflavonoids contained in ginkgo are extremely powerful antioxidants and help combat fatigue by improving circulation to the brain. They also appear to have a strong affinity for the adrenal and thyroid glands and may boost function in these essential glands.

Herbs for Menopause and PMS

Many plants can be useful in the treatment of both PMS and menopause because they actually contain small amounts of the female hormones estrogen and progesterone. These plants, called phytoestrogens, include the following:

Bioflavonoid-Containing Plants. Bioflavonoids were discussed in the vitamin section; in their purified form, they help relieve symptoms of estrogen imbalance and deficiency as well as heavy menstrual flow. However, some women may want to use the actual plant sources of the bioflavonoids as part of their nutritional program. This approach has some benefits because whole plant extracts often contain a wide range of useful nutrients that support the therapeutic effects of the bioflavonoids themselves. As mentioned earlier, bioflavonoids occur in a large variety of fruits and flowers. Excellent sources include citrus fruits, cherry, grape, and hawthorn berry. According to research studies, they have also been found in red clover and subterranean clover strains in Australia. All of these plants are available in capsule or tincture form for women wanting to use them as herbal supplements.

Many medical studies of citrus bioflavonoids have demonstrated their usefulness in treating menopause-related hot flashes and insomnia. They are also useful in controlling menopause-related anxiety and mood swings because they have weak estrogenic activity (1/50,000 the strength of a drug dose of estrogen). Plants containing bioflavonoids may be particularly useful for women who cannot or do not choose to use standard estrogen replacement therapy. This is often the case in women with preexisting health problems like breast or uterine cancer, hypotension, or blood clots. In addition, women who have already experienced side effects from estrogen such as bloating, breast tenderness, or even a worsening of anxiety symptoms or mood swings may not wish to continue on prescription estrogen. The very low potency of bioflavonoids make them ideal nutrients for menopause because the risk of side effects is minimal.

Because bioflavonoids are also antiestrogenic, herbs containing high levels of this nutrient are useful in stabilizing mood and reducing anxiety in my PMS patients. PMS mood symptoms can be linked in some women to an estrogen-progesterone imbalance. Both of these hormones affect brain chemistry and mood. Progesterone has a sedative-like effect while estrogen in excess can worsen anxiety symptoms. Thus, the proper balance between the two female hormones is quite important.

Other Phytoestrogens. Other phytoestrogen plant sources of estrogen and progesterone used in traditional herbology for menopause symptoms include dong quai, black cohosh, blue cohosh, unicorn root, false unicorn root, fennel, anise, sarsaparilla, and wild yam root. The hormonal activities of these plants have been observed in a number of interesting research studies.

Plants may also form the basis for the production of medical hormones. Many common plants such as soy beans and yams contain a preformed steroidal nucleus. Estrogen and progesterone can be synthesized from plants in relatively few steps and have allowed prescription female sex hormones to become widely commercially available.

Herbs for Food Allergies and Hypoglycemia

Many herbs can be used to help the digestive process and stabilize the blood sugar level. These include the following:

Herbal Digestive Aids. Many herbs reduce symptoms of food intolerance such as bloating, abdominal cramps, diarrhea, constipation, fatigue, headache, and mood swings by improving the digestive process. They do this by aiding in the more efficient breakdown of food to basic constituents (amino acids, fatty acids, simple sugars, etc.) and by improving the absorption and assimilation of foods.

Papaya leaf contains powerful enzymes—papain and chymopapain—that help digest protein. These enzymes promote food digestion in women with liver or pancreatic-related health problems. The enzymes in papaya leaf (or the whole papaya fruit itself) make it an important ingredient in dozens of commercial digestive aids. Though papaya leaf has no direct effect on hypoglycemia, it does indirectly help stabilize the blood sugar level by helping break down complex protein- and carbohydrate-containing foods, making their nutrients more available.

Ginger also helps improve digestion and assimilation of foods from the digestive tract into the general circulation. It does this by promoting better blood circulation to the digestive tract, by relaxing smooth muscles in the intestines, and by stimulating the metabolism. Ginger also reduces symptoms of nausea. Like papaya leaf, it has an indirect effect on stabilizing the blood sugar level by helping to increase the availability of essential nutrients through more efficient digestive processes.

Peppermint and fennel also help to calm upset stomach, normalize bowel function, and eliminate heartburn and intestinal spasm. Peppermint also has anti-inflammatory and anti-infective properties that can help promote healthier intestinal absorption and assimilation. Peppermint (and other members of the mint family) have been found in research studies to have potent antiviral, antibacterial, and antifungal effects. Garlic is another powerful herb that helps to normalize the digestive process by inhibiting pathological micro-organisms such as fungi, viruses, and bacteria, and promoting the growth of beneficial flora. It is particularly useful in the suppression of intestinal candida. Overgrowth of a pathogenic fungus, candida albicans, can cause a variety of unpleasant digestive symptoms.

Blood Sugar Stabilizers. Several herbs have been found to stabilize the blood sugar level, thereby reducing or eliminating the mood swings and symptoms of hypoglycemia.

Most prominent among these herbs is Siberian ginseng. This herb is an adaptogen, which helps to protect the body against the effects of both physical and mental stress. It has a normalizing effect on the blood sugar level, raising it when it falls too low and decreasing it when it becomes abnormally high. Siberian ginseng also helps reduce anxiety and mood swings by its ability to improve adrenal function, thus protecting the body from the harmful effects of stress. The use of Siberian ginseng allows people to withstand increased workloads, exercise levels, and noise, among other stress factors. It also improves mental alertness and energy levels and helps decrease fatigue in women with anxiety symptoms. The effects of Siberian ginseng build up over time;

therefore, you may need to use it for several weeks to months before experiencing symptom relief.

Gotu kola helps to stabilize the blood sugar level by improving adrenal function. It behaves similarly to Siberian ginseng, acting as a potent antifatigue nutrient. Women who are experiencing excessive levels of anxiety may find the energy-supporting qualities of both these herbs to be quite helpful during stressful periods.

Sedative and Relaxant Herbs

Balm
Bay
Catnip
Celery
Hops
Motherwort

Blood Circulation Enhancers

Ginger

Chronic Fatigue and Depression

Dandelion root
Ginger
Ginkgo biloba

Phytoestrogens and Progesterone-like Herbs

Anise
Black cohosh
Blue cohosh
Citrus fruits
Cherry
Dong quai

Herbal Digestants

Fennel
Garlic
Ginger

Blood Sugar Stabilizers

Siberian ginseng
Gotu kola

Essential Fatty Acids for Relief of Anxiety

Essential fatty acids are an extremely important part of the nutritional program for any women with anxiety and stress symptoms. Essential fatty acids are the raw materials from which the beneficial hormone-like chemicals called prostaglandins are made. Prostaglandins have muscle-relaxant and blood-vessel-relaxant properties that can significantly reduce muscle cramps and tension. They also have a calming and relaxing effect on the emotions. Because of their beneficial effects, they have been used in the treatment of PMS, anxiety, eating disorders, and menopause.

Linoleic acid (Omega 6 family) and linolenic acid (Omega-3 family), the two essential fatty acids, are derived from specific food sources in our diet, primarily raw seeds and nuts, and certain fish including salmon, mackerel, and trout. Linoleic and linolenic acids are not made by the body and must be supplied daily in our diets, through either food or supplements. Even if the diet contains significant fatty acids, some women may lack the ability to convert them efficiently to the muscle-relaxant prostaglandins. This is particularly true of linoleic acid, which must be converted to a chemical called gamma linolenic acid (GLA) on its way to becoming the series-one prostaglandin.

The conversion of linoleic acid to GLA, followed by the chemical steps leading to the creation of the beneficial prostaglandins, requires the presence of magnesium, vitamin B_6, zinc, vitamin C, and niacin. Women deficient in these nutrients can't make the chemical conversions effectively. In addition, women who eat a high-cholesterol diet, eat processed oils such as mayonnaise, use a great deal of alcohol, or are diabetic may find the fatty acid conversion to the series-one prostaglandin difficult to achieve. Other factors that impede prostaglandin production include emotional stress, allergies, and eczema. In women with these risk factors, less than 1 percent of linoleic acid may be converted to GLA. The rest of the fatty acids may be used as an energy source, but they will not be able to play a role in relieving anxiety and stress symptoms.

The best food sources of essential fatty acids are raw flax seed oil and pumpkin seed oil, which contain high levels of both fatty acids, linoleic and linolenic. Both the seeds and their pressed oils can be used and should be absolutely fresh and unspoiled. As mentioned earlier, these oils become rancid very easily when exposed to light and air (oxygen), and they need to be packed in special opaque containers and kept in the refrigerator.

My special favorite is fresh flax seed oil; golden, rich and delicious. It is extremely high in linoleic and linolenic acids, which comprise approximately 80 percent of its total content. Flax oil has a wonderful flavor and can be used as a butter replacement on foods such as mashed potatoes, air-popped popcorn, steamed broccoli, cauliflower, carrots, and bread. Flax oil (and all other essential oils) should never be heated or used in cooking, as heat affects the special chemical properties of these oils. Instead, add these oils as a flavoring to foods that are already cooked. Pumpkin seed oil has a deep green color and spicy flavor, and is probably more difficult to find than flax seed oil. Fresh raw pumpkin seeds are a good source of this oil. Usually available at health food stores, both flax seed oil and pumpkin seed oil can also be taken in capsule form.

Linolenic acid (Omega-3 family) is found in abundance in fish oils. The best sources are cold-water, high-fat fish such as salmon, tuna, rainbow trout, mackerel, and eel. Linoleic acid (Omega-6 family) is found in many seeds and seed oils. Good sources include safflower oil, sunflower oil, corn oil, sesame seed oil, and wheat germ oil. Many women prefer to use fresh raw sesame seeds, sunflower seeds, and wheat germ to obtain the oils.

The average healthy adult requires only four teaspoons per day of the essential oils. However, women with anxiety and stress symptoms who may have a real deficiency of these oils need up to two or three tablespoons per day until their symptoms improve. Occasionally, these oils may cause diarrhea; if this occurs, use only one teaspoon per day. Women with acne and very oily skin should use them cautiously. For optimal results, be sure to use these oils along with vitamin E.

How to Use Vitamins, Minerals, and Herbal Supplements

Good dietary habits are crucial for relief of anxiety and stress-related symptoms, but many women must also use nutritional supplements to achieve high levels of certain essential nutrients. This section contains formulas that you can use to treat anxiety related to different causes. I have included both vitamin and mineral formulas and herbal formulas so that you will have a wide range of supplements from which to chose.

I recommend that women with anxiety take supplements cautiously. Start with one-quarter of the daily dose listed in the following formulas. Do not go to a higher dose level unless you are sure you can tolerate the dose you're already using.

I recommend that all supplements be taken with meals or at least with a snack. A digestive reaction to supplements, such as nausea or indigestion, is rare. If this happens to you, stop all supplements and start them again one at a time until you find the offending nutrient. Any nutrient to which you have a reaction should be eliminated from your program. If you have any specific questions about nutritional supplementation, be sure to ask your physician.

Nutritional System for Anxiety, Panic, Food Addictions, and Anxiety Coexisting with Depression or Mitral Valve Prolapse

Vitamins and Minerals	Maximum Daily Dose
Beta carotene (provitamin A)	25,000 I.U.
Vitamin B complex	
B_1 (thiamine)	50–100 mg
B_2 (riboflavin)	50–100 mg
B_3 (niacinamide)	50–100 mg
B_5 (pantothenic acid)	50–200 mg
B_6 (pyridoxine)	50–200 mg
B_{12} (cyanocobalamin)	100 mcg
Folic acid	400 mcg
Biotin	400 mcg
Choline	250–500 mg
Inositol	250–500 mg
PABA (para-aminobenzoic acid)	50–100 mg
Vitamin C	2000–5000 mg
Vitamin D	400 I.U.
Vitamin E (d-alpha tocopherol acetate)	400–800 I.U.
Calcium aspartate	500–1000 mg
Magnesium aspartate	250–500 mg
Potassium aspartate	100–200 mg
Iron	18 mg
Chromium	150 mcg
Manganese	20 mg
Selenium	50 mcg
Zinc	15 mg
Copper	2 mg
Iodine	150 mcg

Dosage: Take one-quarter to full amount of the above nutrients on a daily basis. Begin this formula with the lowest dose of each nutrient and increase the dose slowly and gradually to the recommended maximum, depending on how you are feeling.

Herbal-based Nutritional System for Anxiety, Panic, Food Addictions, and Anxiety Coexisting with Depression or Mitral Valve Prolapse

(Note: Formula also contains vitamins and minerals in small amounts).

Nutrient	Potency
Vitamin B complex	
B_1 (thiamine)	1.5 mg
B_2 (riboflavin)	1.7 mg
B_3 (niacinamide)	20 mg
B_5 (pantothenic acid)	50 mg
B_6 (pyridoxine)	5 mg
B_{12} (cyanocobalamin)	10 mcg
Folic acid	400 mcg
Biotin	300 mcg
Choline	50 mg
Inositol	150 mg
PABA (para-aminobenzoic acid)	5 mg
Calcium	150 mg
Magnesium	75 mg
Passionflower	50 mg
Valerian root	50 mg
Chamomile	50 mg
Catnip	30 mg
Skullcap	25 mg
Celery	25 mg

Dosage: Take one-half to full amount of the above nutrients before going to bed at night or as needed (not to exceed double the full dose in a four- to six-hour period) during times of stress.

Optimal Nutritional Supplementation for Anxiety Related to PMS, Hypoglycemia, and Hyperthyroidism

Vitamins and Minerals	Maximum Daily Dose
Beta carotene (provitamin A)	15,000 I.U.
Vitamin B complex	
B_1 (thiamine)	50 mg
B_2 (riboflavin)	50 mg
B_3 (niacinamide)	50 mg
B_5 (pantothenic acid)	50 mg
B_6 (pyridoxine)	300 mcg
B_{12} (cyanocobalamin)	50 mcg
Folic acid	200 mcg
Biotin	30 mcg
Choline bitartrate	500 mg
Inositol	500 mg
PABA (para-aminobenzoic acid)	50 mg
Vitamin C	1000 mg
Vitamin D	100 I.U.
Vitamin E	600 I.U.
Calcium	150 mg
Magnesium	300 mg
Iodine	150 mcg
Iron	15 mg
Copper	0.5 mg
Zinc	25 mg
Manganese	10 mg
Potassium	100 mg
Selenium	25 mcg
Chromium	100 mcg

Dosage: Take one-quarter to full amount of the above nutrients on a daily basis. Begin this formula with the lowest dose of each nutrient and increase the dose slowly and gradually to the recommended maximum, depending on how you are feeling.

Herbs (as capsules)	Maximum Daily Dose
Burdock	210 mg
Sarsaparilla	210 mg
Ginger	70 mg

Dosage: Take one to two capsules per day.

Optimal Nutritional Supplementation for Anxiety Related to Menopause

Vitamins and Minerals	Maximum Daily Dose
Beta carotene	5000 I.U.
Vitamin A	5000 I.U.
Vitamin D	400 I.U.
Vitamin E (d-alpha tocopherol acetate)	800 I.U.
Vitamin C	1000 mg
Bioflavonoids	800 mg
Rutin	200 mg
Vitamin B_1	50 mg
Vitamin B_2	50 mg
Vitamin B_3 (Niacin—as niacinamide)	50 mg
Vitamin B_5 (Pantothenic acid)	50 mg
Vitamin B_6	30 mg
Vitamin B_{12}	50 mcg
Folic acid	400 mcg
Biotin	200 mcg
Choline	50 mg
Inositol	50 mg
PABA (para-aminobenzoic acid)	50 mg
Calcium (calcium citrate)	1200 mg
Magnesium	320 mg
Iodine	150 mcg
Iron (ferrous fumarate)	27 mg
Copper	2 mg

Vitamins and Minerals	Maximum Daily Dose
Zinc	15 mg
Manganese	10 mg
Potassium (potassium aspartate)	100 mg
Selenium	25 mcg
Chromium	100 mcg
Bromelain	100 mg
Papain	65 mg
Boron	3 mg

Dosage: Women with mild to moderate menopause symptoms can use the formula at half strength. Women with severe symptoms should use the full strength.

Herbs (as capsules)	Maximum Daily Dose
Fennel	100 mg
Anise	100 mg
Blessed thistle	100 mg
False unicorn root	100 mg
Blue cohosh	100 mg

Dosage: Take one to two capsules per day.

Food Sources of Vitamin A

Vegetables	Fruits	Meat, Poultry, Seafood
Carrots	Apricots	Crab
Carrot juice	Avocado	Halibut
Collard greens	Cantaloupe	Liver—all types
Dandelion greens	Mangoes	Mackerel
Green onion	Papaya	Salmon
Kale	Peaches	Swordfish
Parsley	Persimmons	
Spinach		
Sweet potatoes		
Turnip greens		
Winter squash		

Food Sources of Vitamin B Complex

Vegetables and Legumes
Alfalfa
Artichokes
Asparagus
Beets
Broccoli
Brussels sprouts
Cabbage
Cauliflower
Corn
Garbanzo beans
Green beans
Green peas
Kale
Leeks
Lentils
Lima beans
Onions
Pinto beans
Romaine lettuce
Soybeans

Meat, Poultry, Seafood
Egg yolks*
Liver*

Grains
Barley
Bran
Brown rice
Corn
Millet
Rice bran
Wheat
Wheat germ

Sweeteners
Blackstrap molasses

Eggs and meat should be from organic free-range stock fed on pesticide-free food.

Food Sources of Vitamin B₆

Grains
Brown rice
Buckwheat flour
Rice bran
Rice polishings
Rye flour
Wheat germ
Whole wheat flour

Vegetables
Asparagus
Beet greens
Broccoli
Brussels sprouts
Cauliflower
Green peas
Leeks
Sweet potatoes

Meat, Poultry, Seafood
Chicken
Salmon
Shrimp
Tuna

Nuts and Seeds
Sunflower seeds

Food Sources of Vitamin C

Fruits	Vegetables	Meat, Poultry, Seafood
Blackberries	Asparagus	Liver—all types
Black currants	Black-eyed peas	Pheasant
Cantaloupe	Broccoli	Quail
Elderberries	Brussels sprouts	Salmon
Grapefruit	Cabbage	
Grapefruit juice	Cauliflower	
Guavas	Collards	
Kiwi fruit	Green onions	
Mangoes	Green peas	
Oranges	Kale	
Orange juice	Kohlrabi	
Pineapple	Parsley	
Raspberries	Potatoes	
Strawberries	Rutabaga	
Tangerines	Sweet pepper	
	Sweet potatoes	
	Tomatoes	
	Turnips	

Food Sources of Vitamin E

Vegetables
Asparagus
Cucumber
Green peas
Kale

Nuts and Seeds
Almonds
Brazil nuts
Hazelnuts
Peanuts

Meat, Poultry, Seafood
Haddock
Herring
Lamb
Liver—all types
Mackerel

Fruits
Mangoes

Oils
Corn oil
Peanut oil
Safflower oil
Sesame oil
Soybean oil
Wheat germ oil

Grains
Brown rice
Millet

Food Sources of Essential Fatty Acids

Flax oil
Pumpkin oil
Soybean oil
Walnut oil
Safflower oil

Sunflower oil
Grape oil
Corn oil
Wheat germ oil
Sesame oil

Food Sources of Calcium

Vegetables and Legumes
Artichoke
Black beans
Black-eyed peas
Beet greens
Broccoli
Brussels sprouts
Cabbage
Collards
Eggplant
Garbanzo beans
Green beans
Green onions
Kale
Kidney beans
Leeks
Lentils
Parsley
Parsnips
Pinto beans
Rutabaga
Soybeans
Spinach
Turnips
Watercress

Meat, Poultry, and Seafood
Abalone
Beef
Bluefish
Carp
Crab
Haddock
Herring
Lamb
Lobster
Oysters
Perch
Salmon
Shrimp
Venison

Fruits and Juices
Blackberries
Black currants
Boysenberries
Oranges
Pineapple juice
Prunes
Raisins
Rhubarb
Tangerine juice

Grains
Bran
Brown rice
Bulgar wheat
Millet

Food Sources of Magnesium

Vegetables and Legumes
Artichokes
Black-eyed peas
Carrot juice
Corn
Green peas
Leeks
Lima beans
Okra
Parsnips
Potatoes
Soybean sprouts
Spinach
Squash
Yams

Nuts and Seeds
Almonds
Brazil nuts
Hazelnuts
Peanuts
Pistachios
Pumpkin seeds
Sesame seeds
Walnuts

Fruits and Juices
Avocados
Bananas
Grapefruit juice
Papayas
Pineapple juice
Prunes
Raisins

Grains
Brown rice
Millet
Wild rice

Meat, Poultry, Seafood
Beef
Carp
Chicken
Clams
Cod
Crab
Duck
Haddock
Herring
Lamb
Mackerel
Oysters
Salmon
Shrimp
Snapper
Turkey

Food Sources of Zinc

Grains	Vegetables and Legumes	Fruits
Barley	Black-eyed peas	Apples
Brown rice	Cabbage	Peaches
Buckwheat	Carrots	
Corn	Garbanzo beans	**Meat, Poultry, Seafood**
Cornmeal	Green peas	
Millet	Lentils	Chicken
Oatmeal	Lettuce	Oysters
Rice bran	Lima beans	
Rye bread	Onions	
Wheat bran	Soy flour	
Wheat germ	Soy meal	
Wheat berries	Soy protein	
Whole wheat bread		
Whole wheat flour		

6

Relaxation Techniques for Relief of Anxiety & Stress

Women with increased levels of anxiety and nervous tension often need to develop more effective ways of dealing with day-to-day stresses—the minor everyday pressures that women with a healthy emotional balance handle easily but that can be overwhelming for women whose anxiety responses are easily triggered. Such stress can include riding in an elevator, being in crowds, going to the dentist, or any situation, place, or person that sparks a woman's emotional charge. Often these charged issues evoke anxiety, fear, or upset feelings. Moreover, significant lifestyle changes—death of a loved one, divorce, job loss, financial problems, major changes in personal relationships—can be almost impossible to handle when a woman is already feeling anxious and tense. Being unable to cope with stress effectively can also damage a woman's self-esteem and self-confidence. A woman with anxiety episodes may feel a decreasing sense of self-worth as her ability to handle her usual range of activities diminishes. Life stresses themselves don't necessarily change, so how a woman copes with them can really make the difference.

How Stress Affects the Body

Your emotional and physical reactions to stress are partly determined by the sensitivity of your sympathetic nervous system. This system produces the fight-or-flight reaction in response to stress and excitement, speeding up and heightening the pulse rate, respiration, muscle tension, glandular function, and circulation of the blood. If you have recurrent anxiety symptoms, either major or minor lifestyle and emotional upsets may cause an overreaction of your sympathetic system. If you have an especially stressful life, your sympathetic nervous system may always be poised to react to a crisis, putting you in a state of constant tension. In this mode, you tend to react to small stresses the same way you would react to real emergencies. The energy that accumulates in the body to meet this "emergency" must be discharged in order to bring your body back into balance. Repeated episodes of the fight-or-flight reaction deplete your energy reserves and, if they continue, cause a downward spiral that can lead to emotional burnout and eventually complete exhaustion. You can break this spiral only by learning to manage stress in a way that protects and even increases your energy level.

Techniques for Relaxation

Many patients have asked me about techniques for coping more effectively with stress. Although I send some women for counseling or psychotherapy when symptoms are severe, most are looking for practical ways to manage stress on their own. They want to take responsibility for handling their own problems—observing their inadequate methods of dealing with stress, learning new techniques to improve their habits, and then practicing these techniques on a regular basis.

I have included relaxation and stress reduction exercises in many of my patient programs. The feedback has been very positive; many patients report an increased sense of well-being from these self help techniques. They also note an improvement in their physical health. This chapter includes fourteen stress-reduction exercises for women with anxiety. They will take you through a series of specific steps to help alleviate your symptoms. The exercises will teach you the following helpful techniques: focusing and meditation, grounding techniques (how to feel more centered), exercises that help you to relax and release muscle tension, erasure techniques (how to erase old programs), healing the inner child, visualizations, and affirmations. These techniques will help you cope with stress more efficiently, make your thoughts more calm and peaceful, and help you learn to relax, while you build self-esteem and self-confidence. Try them all; then decide which ones produce the greatest benefits for you. Practice these on a regular basis.

Quieting the Mind and Body

Women with recurring symptoms of anxiety and nervous tension are usually barraged by a constant stream of negative "self-talk." Throughout the day your conscious mind may be inundated with thoughts, feelings, and fantasies that trigger feelings of upset. Many of these thoughts replay unresolved issues of health, finances, or personal and work relationships. This relentless mental replay of unresolved issues can reinforce the anxiety symptoms and be exhausting. It is important to know how to shut off the constant inner dialogue and quiet the mind.

The first two exercises require you to sit quietly and engage in a simple repetitive activity. By emptying your mind, you give yourself a rest. Meditation allows you to create a state of deep relaxation, which is very healing to the entire body. Metabolism slows, as do physiological functions such as heart rate and blood pressure. Muscle tension decreases. Brain wave patterns shift from the fast beta waves that occur during a normal active day to the slower alpha waves, which appear just before falling asleep or in times of deep relaxation. If you practice these exercises regularly, they can help relieve anxiety by resting your mind and turning off upsetting thoughts.

Exercise 1: Focusing

Select a small personal object that you like a great deal. It might be a jeweled pin or a simple flower from your garden. Focus all your attention on this object as you inhale and exhale slowly and deeply for one to two minutes. While you are doing this exercise, try not to let any other thoughts or feelings enter your mind. If they do, just return your attention to the object. At the end of this exercise you will probably feel more peaceful and calmer. Any tension or nervousness that you were feeling upon starting the exercise should be diminished.

Exercise 2: Meditation

- Sit or lie in a comfortable position.

- Close your eyes and breathe deeply. Let your breathing be slow and relaxed.

- Focus all your attention on your breathing. Notice the movement of your chest and abdomen in and out.

- Block out all other thoughts, feelings, and sensations. If you feel your attention wandering, bring it back to your breathing.

- As you inhale, say the word "peace" to yourself, and as you exhale, say the word "calm." Draw out the pronunciation of the word so that it lasts for the entire breath. The word "peace" sounds like p-e-e-a-a-a-c-c-c-e-e-e. The word "calm" sounds like: c-a-a-a-l-l-l-l-m-m-m. Repeating these words as you breathe will help you to concentrate.

- Continue this exercise until you feel very relaxed.

Grounding Techniques

Many women suffering from anxiety episodes often feel ungrounded and disorganized. There is a pervasive sense of "things falling apart." When anxiety episodes occur, it often takes a concentrated effort just to get through the day, accomplishing such basic daily tasks as cooking, housecleaning, taking care of children, or getting to work or school. The next two exercises teach you grounding techniques that will help you feel more centered and focused. Practicing either of these exercises will allow you to organize your energies and proceed more effectively with your daily routine.

Exercise 3: Oak Tree Meditation

- Sit in a comfortable position, your arms resting at your sides.

- Close your eyes and breathe deeply. Let your breathing be slow and relaxed.

- See your body as a strong oak tree. Your body is solid like the wide, brown trunk of the tree. Imagine sturdy roots growing from your legs and going down deeply into the earth, anchoring your body. You feel solid and strong, able to handle any stress.

- When upsetting thoughts or situations occur, visualize your body remaining grounded like the oak tree. Feel the strength and stability in your arms and legs.

- You feel confident and relaxed, able to handle any situation.

Exercise 4: Grounding Cord Meditation

- Sit in a comfortable position, your arms resting comfortably at your sides.

- Close your eyes and breathe deeply. Let your breathing be slow and relaxed.

- Imagine a thick wide cord attaching itself to the base of your spine. This is your grounding cord. It can be a thick piece of rope, a tree trunk, or any other material that feels strong and stable.

Make sure your cord is wide and sturdy enough. Then imagine a thick metal hook attaching itself to the end of your cord.

- Now visualize your grounding cord dropping down two hundred feet below the earth and hooking on to the solid bedrock below the earth.

- Continue to breathe deeply and notice the sense of peace and stability that your grounding cord can bring you.

- Replace the cord with a new one each day or whenever you feel your emotions getting out of control.

Releasing Muscle Tension

The next three exercises will help you get in touch with your areas of muscle tension and then help you learn to release this tension. This is an important sequence for women with emotional symptoms of anxiety and nervous tension since habitual emotional patterns cause certain muscle groups to tense and tighten. For example, if a person has difficulty in expressing feelings, the neck muscles may be chronically tense. A person with a lot of repressed anger may have chest pain and tight chest muscles. Contracted muscles limit movement and energy flow in the body, since they tend to have decreased blood circulation and oxygenation and accumulate an excess of waste products, such as carbon dioxide and lactic acid. Therefore, muscle tension can be a significant cause of the fatigue that often accompanies chronic stress. The following exercises help release tension and the blocked emotions held in tight muscles.

Exercise 5: Discovering Muscle Tension

- Lie on your back in a comfortable position. Allow your arms to rest at your sides, palms down, on the surface next to you.

- Raise just the right hand and arm and hold it elevated for 15 seconds.

- Notice if your forearm feels tight and tense or if the muscles are soft and pliable.

- Let your hand and arm drop down and relax. The arm muscles will relax too.

- As you lie still, notice any other parts of your body that feel tense, muscles that feel tight and sore. You may notice a constant dull aching in certain muscles.

Exercise 6: Progressive Muscle Relaxation

- Lie on your back in a comfortable position. Allow your arms to rest at your sides, palms down, on the surface next to you.

- Inhale and exhale slowly and deeply.

- Clench your hands into fists and hold them tightly for 15 seconds. As you do this, relax the rest of your body. Visualize your fists contracting, becoming tighter and tighter.

- Then let your hands relax. On relaxing, see a golden light flowing into the entire body, making all your muscles soft and pliable.

- Now, tense and relax the following parts of your body in this order: face, shoulders, back, stomach, pelvis, legs, feet, and toes. Hold each part tensed for 15 seconds and then relax your body for 30 seconds before going on to the next part.

- Finish the exercise by shaking your hands and imagining the remaining tension flowing out of your fingertips.

Exercise 7: Release of Muscle Tension and Anxiety

- Lie in a comfortable position. Allow your arms to rest at your sides, palms down. Inhale and exhale slowly and deeply with your eyes closed.

- Become aware of your feet, ankles, and legs. Notice if these parts of your body have any muscle tension or tightness. If so, how does the tense part of your body feel? Is it viselike, knotted, cold, numb? Do you notice any strong feelings, such as hurt, upset, or anger, in that part of your body? Breathe into that part of your body until you feel it relax. Release any anxious feelings with your breathing, continuing until they begin to decrease in intensity and fade.

- Next, move your awareness into your hips, pelvis, and lower back. Note any tension there. Notice any anxious feelings located in that part of your body. Breathe into your hips and pelvis until you feel them relax. Release any negative emotions as you breathe in and out.

- Focus on your abdomen and chest. Notice any anxious feelings located in this area and let them drop away as you breathe in and out. Continue to release any upsetting feelings located in your abdomen or chest.

- Finally, focus on your head, neck, arms, and hands. Note any tension in this area and release it. With your breathing, release any negative feelings blocked in this area until you can't feel them anymore.

- When you have finished releasing tension throughout the body, continue deep breathing and relaxing for another minute or two. At the end of this exercise, you should feel lighter and more energized.

Erasing Stress and Tension

Often the situations and beliefs that make us feel anxious and tense look large and insurmountable. We tend to form representations in our mind that empower stress. In these representations, we look tiny and helpless, while the stressors look huge and unsolvable. You can change these mental representations and cut stressors down to size. The next two exercises will help you to gain mastery over stress by learning to shrink it or even erase it with your mind. This places stress in a much more manageable and realistic perspective. These two exercises will also help engender a sense of power and mastery, thereby reducing anxiety and restoring a sense of calm.

Exercise 8: Shrinking Stress

- Sit or lie in a comfortable position. Breathe slowly and deeply.

- Visualize a situation, person, or even a belief (such as, "I'm afraid of the dark" or "I don't want to give that public speech") that makes you feel anxious and tense.

- As you do this, you might see a person's face, a place you're afraid to go, or simply a dark cloud. Where do you see this stressful picture? Is it above you, to one side, or in front of you? How does it look? Is it big or little, dark or light? Does it have certain colors?

- Now slowly begin to shrink the stressful picture. Continue to see the stressful picture shrinking until it is so small that it can literally be held in the palm of your hand. Hold your hand out in front of you, and place the picture in the palm of your hand.

- If the stressor has a characteristic sound (like a voice or traffic noise), hear it getting tiny and soft. As it continues to shrink, its voice or sounds become almost inaudible.

- Now the stressful picture is so small it can fit on your second finger. Watch it shrink from there until it finally turns into a little dot and disappears.

- Often this exercise causes feelings of amusement, as well as relaxation, as the feared stressor shrinks, gets less intimidating, and finally disappears.

Exercise 9: Erasing Stress

- Sit or lie in a comfortable position. Breathe slowly and deeply.

- Visualize a situation, a person, or even a belief (such as, "I'm afraid to go to the shopping mall" or "I'm scared to mix with other people at parties") that causes you to feel anxious and fearful.

- As you do this you might see a specific person, an actual place, or simply shapes and colors. Where do you see this stressful picture? Is it below you, to the side, in front of you? How does it look? Is it big or little, dark or light, or does it have a specific color?

- Imagine that a large eraser, like the kind used to erase chalk marks, has just floated into your hand. Actually feel and see the eraser in your hand. Take the eraser and begin to rub it over the area where the stressful picture is located. As the eraser rubs out the stressful picture it fades, shrinks, and finally disappears. When you can no longer see the stressful picture, simply continue to focus on your deep breathing for another minute, inhaling and exhaling slowly and deeply.

Healing the Inner Child

Many of our anxieties and fears come from our inner child rather than our adult self. Sometimes it is difficult to realize that the emotional upsets we feel are actually feelings left over from childhood fears, traumas, and experiences. When unhealed, they remain with us into adulthood, causing emotional distress over issues that competent "grown-up" people feel they should be able to handle. For example, fear of the dark, fear of being unlovable, and fear of rejection often originate in early dysfunctional or unhappy experiences with our parents and siblings. While many of these deep, unresolved emotional issues may require counseling, particularly if they are causing anxiety episodes, there is much that we can do for ourselves to heal childhood wounds. The next exercise helps you to get in touch with your own inner child and facilitates the healing process.

Exercise 10: Healing the Inner Child

- Sit or lie in a comfortable position. Breathe slowly and deeply.

- Begin to get in touch with where your inner child resides. Is she located in your abdomen, in your chest, or by your side? (This may actually be the part of your body where you feel the most fear and anxiety, such as your chest or your pelvis.) How old is she? Can you see what clothes she is wearing? What are her emotions? Is she upset, anxious, sad, or angry? Is she withdrawn and quiet?

- Begin to see her upset feelings flow out of her body and into a container on the floor. Watch the upset feelings wash out of every part of her body until they are all gone and the container is full. Then seal the container and slowly watch it fade and dissolve until it disappears completely, carrying all the upset feelings with it.

- Now begin to fill your inner child with a peaceful, healing, golden light. Watch her become peaceful and mellow as the light fills every cell in her body. Watch her body relax. Give her a toy animal or a doll or even cuddle her in your arms.

- As you leave your inner child feeling peaceful, return your focus to your breathing. Spend a minute inhaling and exhaling deeply and slowly. If you like working with your inner child, return to visit her often!

Visualization

The next two exercises use visualization as a therapeutic method to affect the physical and mental processes of the body; both focus on color. Color therapy, as it applies to human health, has a long and distinguished history. In many studies, scientists have exposed subjects to specific colors, either directly through exposure to light therapy, or through changing the color of their environment. Scientific research throughout the world has shown that color therapy can have a profound effect on health and well-being. It can stimulate the endocrine glands, the immune system, and the nervous system, and help to balance the emotions. Visualizing color in a specific part of the body can have a powerful therapeutic effect, too, and can be a good stress management technique for relief of anxiety and nervous tension.

The first exercise uses the color blue, which provides a calming and relaxing effect. For women with anxiety who are carrying a lot of physical and emotional tension, blue lessens the fight-or-flight response. Blue also calms such physiological functions as pulse rate, breathing, and perspiration, and relaxes the mood. If you experience chronic fatigue and are tense, anxious, or irritable, or carry a lot of muscle tension, the first exercise will be very helpful.

The second exercise uses the color red, which can benefit women who have fatigue due to chronic anxiety and upset. Red stimulates all the endocrine glands, including the pituitary and adrenal glands. It heightens senses such as smell and taste. Emotionally, red is linked to vitality and high energy states. Even though the color red can speed up autonomic nervous system function, women with anxiety-related fatigue can benefit from visualizing this color. I often do the red visualization when I am tired and need a pick-me-up. You may find that you are attracted to the color in one exercise more than another. Use the exercise with the color that appeals to you the most.

Exercise 11: Tension Release Through Color

- Sit or lie in a comfortable position, your arms resting at your sides. As you take a deep breath, visualize that the earth below you is filled with the color blue. This blue color extends 50 feet below you into the earth. Now imagine that you are opening up energy centers on the bottom of your feet. As you inhale, visualize the soft blue color filling up your feet. When your feet are completely filled with the color blue, then bring the color up through your ankles, legs, pelvis, and lower back.

- Each time you exhale, see the blue color leaving through your lungs, carrying any tension and stress with it. See the tension dissolve into the air.

- Continue to inhale blue into your abdomen, chest, shoulders, arms, neck, and head. Exhale the blue slowly out of your lungs. Repeat this entire process five times and then relax for a few minutes.

Exercise 12: Energizing Through Color

- Sit or lie in a comfortable position, your arms resting easily at your sides. As you take a deep breath, visualize a big balloon above your head filled with a bright red healing energy. Imagine that you pop this balloon so all the bright red energy is released.

- As you inhale, see the bright red color filling up your head. It fills up your brain, your face, and the bones of your skull. Let the bright red color pour in until your head is ready to overflow with color. Then let the red color flow into your neck, shoulders, arms, and chest. As you exhale, breathe the red color out of your lungs, taking any tiredness and fatigue with it. Breathe any feeling of fatigue out of your body.

- As you inhale, continue to bring the bright, energizing red color into your abdomen, pelvis, lower back, legs, and feet until your whole body is filled with red. Exhale the red color out of your lungs, continuing to release any feeling of fatigue. Repeat this process five times. At the end of this exercise, you should feel more energized and vibrant. Your mental energy should feel more vitalized and clear.

Affirmations

The following two exercises give you healthful affirmations that are very useful for women with anxiety. As described earlier, anxiety symptoms are due to a complex interplay between the mind and body. Your state of emotional and physical health is determined in part by the thousands of mental messages you send yourself each day with your thoughts. For example, if fear of public places triggers your anxiety symptoms, the mind will send a constant stream of messages to you reinforcing your beliefs about the dangers and mishaps that can occur in public places. The fright triggers muscle tension and shallow breathing. Similarly, if you constantly criticize the way you look, your lack of self-love may be reflected in your body. For example, your shoulders will slump and you may have a dull and lackluster countenance.

Affirmations provide a method to change these negative belief systems to thoughts that preserve peace and calm. Positive statements replace the anxiety-inducing messages with thoughts that make you feel good.

The first affirmation exercise gives you a series of statements to promote a sense of emotional and physical health and well-being. Using these affirmations may create a feeling of emotional peace by changing your negative beliefs about your body and health into positive beliefs. The second affirmation exercise helps promote self-esteem and self-confidence and also helps to reduce anxiety. Many women with high anxiety lose their self-confidence and feel depressed and defeated by their condition. They feel frustrated and somehow at fault for not finding a solution. Repeat each affirmation to yourself or say them out loud 3 to 5 minutes. Use either or both exercises on a regular basis to promote healthful, positive thought patterns.

Exercise 13: Positive Mind-Body Affirmations

- I handle stress and tension appropriately and effectively.

- My mood is calm and relaxed.

- I can cope well and get on with my life during times of stress.

- I think thoughts that uplift and nurture me.

- I enjoy thinking positive thoughts that make me feel good about myself and my life.

- I deserve to feel good right now.

- I feel peaceful and calm.

- My breathing is slow and calm.

- My muscles are relaxed and comfortable.

- I feel grounded and fully present.

- I can effectively handle any situation that comes my way.

- I think through the solutions to my emotional issues slowly and peacefully.

- I am thankful for all the positive things in my life.

- I practice the relaxation methods that I enjoy.

- My body is healthy and strong.

- I eat a well-balanced and nutritious diet.

- I enjoy eating delicious and healthful food.

- My body wants food that is easy to digest and high in vitamins and minerals.

- I do regular exercise in a relaxed and enjoyable manner.

Exercise 14: Self-Esteem Affirmations

- I am filled with energy, vitality, and self-confidence.

- I am pleased with how I handle my emotional needs.

- I know exactly how to manage my daily schedule to promote my emotional and physical well-being.

- I listen to my body's needs and regulate my activity level to take care of those needs.

- I love and honor my body.

- I fill my mind with positive and self-nourishing thoughts.

- I am a wonderful and worthy person.

- I deserve health, vitality, and peace of mind.

- I have total confidence in my ability to heal myself.

- I feel radiant with abundant energy and vitality.

- The world around me is full of radiant beauty and abundance.

- I am attracted only to those people and situations that support and nurture me.

- I appreciate the positive people and situations that are currently in my life.

- I love and honor myself.

- I enjoy my positive thoughts and feelings.

More Stress-Reduction Techniques for Anxiety

The rest of this chapter contains additional techniques useful for relief of anxiety and relaxation of tight and tense muscles. These methods induce deep emotional relaxation. Try them for a delightful experience.

Hydrotherapy

For centuries, people have used warm water as a way to calm moods and relax muscles. You can have your own "spa" at home by adding relaxing ingredients to the bath water. I have found the following formula to be extremely useful in relieving muscle pain and tension.

Alkaline Bath. Run a tub of warm water. Heat will increase your menstrual flow, so keep the water a little cooler if heavy flow is a problem. Add one cup of sea salt and one cup of bicarbonate of soda to the tub. This is a highly alkaline mixture and I recommend using it only once or twice a month. I've found it very helpful in reducing cramps and calming anxiety and irritability. Soak for 20 minutes. You will probably feel very relaxed and sleepy after this bath; use it at night before going to sleep. You will probably wake up feeling refreshed and energized the following day. Heat of any kind helps to release muscle tension. Many women find that saunas and baths also help to calm their moods.

Sound

Music can have a tremendously relaxing effect on our minds and bodies. For women with anxiety and nervous tension, I recommend slow, quiet music—classical music is particularly good. This type of music can have a pronounced beneficial effect on your physiological functions. It can slow your pulse and heart rate, lower your blood pressure, and decrease your levels of stress hormones. It promotes peace and relaxation and helps to induce sleep. Nature sounds, such as ocean waves and rainfall, can also induce a sense of peace and relaxation. I have patients who keep tapes of nature sounds in their cars and at home for use when they feel more stressed. Play relaxing music often when you are aware of increased emotional and physical tension.

Massage

Massage can be extremely therapeutic for women who feel anxious. Gentle touching either by a trained massage therapist, your relationship partner, or even yourself can be very relaxing. Tension usually fades away relatively quickly with gentle, relaxed touching. The kneading and stroking movement of a good massage relaxes tight muscles and improves circulation. If you can afford to do so, I recommend treating yourself to a professional massage during times of stress. Otherwise, trade with a friend or partner. There are also many books available that instruct people how to massage themselves.

Putting Your Stress-Reduction Program Together

This chapter has introduced you to many different ways to reduce anxiety and stress and make each day calm and peaceful. Try each exercise at least once. Then find the combination that works for you. Doing the exercise you most enjoy should take no longer than 20 to 30 minutes, depending on how much time you wish to spend. Ideally, you should do the exercises daily. Over time, they will help you gain insight into your negative feelings and beliefs while changing them into positive, self-nurturing new ones. Your ability to cope with stress should improve tremendously.

7

Breathing Exercises

Therapeutic breathwork is one of my favorite methods for calming the mood. It can have a major impact on feelings of anxiety and upset. Through the use of controlled breathing exercises, you can lower your anxiety level and generate a feeling of internal peace and calm, as well as relax and loosen your muscles.

When you are breathing slowly and deeply, you take in large amounts of oxygen from the environment. This oxygen is taken into your circulation where it binds to the red blood cells as it travels through the arteries and veins. Oxygen allows the cells to produce and utilize energy and to help remove waste products through the production of carbon dioxide. These waste products are cleared through exhalation by the lungs. Thus, the whole body needs optimal levels of oxygen for its normal cycle of building, repair, and elimination.

When you are in emotional distress, oxygen levels decrease. Breathing tends to become jagged, erratic, and shallow. You may find yourself breathing too fast or you may even stop breathing altogether and hold your breath for prolonged periods of time without realizing it. None of these breathing patterns is healthful. Anxious breathing is often linked to other unhealthy physiological reactions that reflect your body's state of stress. When you are upset and emotionally stressed, you tend to tense and tighten your muscles, constrict blood flow, elevate your pulse rate and heartbeat, and stimulate the output of stressful chemicals from your glands. Waste products such as carbon dioxide and lactic acid also accumulate in your muscles and other tissues.

Therapeutic breathing exercises provide a way to break this pattern and help the mind and body return to a peaceful equilibrium. It is important to do the breathing exercises in a slow and regular manner. First, find a comfortable position. Some exercises you should do lying on your back; for other exercises, you'll sit up, uncross your arms and legs, and keep your back straight.

Exercise 1: Deep Abdominal Breathing

Deep, slow abdominal breathing is a very important technique for the relief of anxiety and stress. It also improves energy and vitality. Abdominal breathing brings adequate oxygen, the fuel for metabolic activity, to all tissues of the body. In contrast, rapid, shallow breathing decreases oxygen supply and keeps you nervous and tense. Deep breathing helps to relax the entire body and strengthens muscles in the chest and abdomen. Do this exercise for 3 to 5 minutes.

- Lie flat on your back with your knees pulled up. Keep your feet slightly apart. Try to breathe in and out through your nose.

- Inhale deeply. As you breathe in, allow your stomach to relax so the air flows into your abdomen. Your stomach should balloon out as you breathe in. Visualize your lungs filling up with air so that your chest swells out.

- Imagine that the air you breathe is filling your body with energy.

- Exhale deeply. As you breathe out, let your stomach and chest collapse. Imagine the air being pushed out, first from your abdomen and then from your lungs.

Exercise 2: Peaceful, Slow Breathing

Breathing slowly and peacefully can decrease anxiety and promote a sense of inner calm. Such breathing helps our mind to slow down and our emotions to become happier and more harmonious. Life feels good. When we are calm, we make better decisions and relate to those around us in a healthier way. Breathing slowly can also calm our physical responses by helping to balance autonomic nervous system function. By slowing down our breathing, we slow down our other physiologic responses. Our muscles relax and our blood vessels dilate; a state of equilibrium is restored.

- Lie flat on your back with your knees pulled up. Keep your feet slightly apart. Try to breathe in and out through your nose.

- Inhale deeply. As you breathe in, allow your stomach to relax so that the air flows into your abdomen. Let your stomach balloon out as you breathe in. Visualize the lowest parts of your lungs filling up with air.

- Imagine that the air you are breathing in is filled with peace and calm; a sensation of peacefulness and calm is filling every cell of your body; your whole body feels warm and relaxed as you breathe in this air. Now, exhale deeply. As you breathe out, imagine the air being pushed out from the bottom of your lungs to the top.

- Repeat this sequence until your entire body feels relaxed and your breathing is slow and regular.

Exercise 3: Grounding Breath

When women are anxious and tense, they often lose a sense of being grounded, literally rooted to the earth. Some women report a sensation of numbness in their legs and feet. They may say that they feel as if they have no legs at all. When we become physically ungrounded by symptoms of emotional distress, it is very difficult to function mentally; we have a hard time focusing and concentrating. We may often have difficulty working through our projects for the day in a coherent manner. This next breathing exercise will help you to ground and focus both physically and mentally. You should feel much more stable and focused by the end of this exercise.

- Sit upright in a chair. Be sure you are in a comfortable position. Keep your feet slightly apart. Try to breathe in and out through your nose.

- Inhale deeply. As you breathe in, allow your stomach to relax so that the air flows into your abdomen. Let your stomach balloon out as you breathe in. Visualize the lowest parts of your lungs filling up with air. Hold your inhalation.

- See a large, thick cord running from the bottom of your buttocks to the center of the earth. Follow the cord all the way down and see it fasten securely to the earth's center. Run two smaller cords from the bottoms of your feet down to the center of the earth also.

- As you exhale, gently push your buttocks into the seat of your chair. Become aware of your buttocks, thighs, calves, ankles, and feet. Feel their strength and solidity.

- Repeat this exercise several times until you feel fully present and grounded.

Exercise 4: Color Breathing with Golden Light

Color breathing has traditionally been used to heal the mind and body and strengthen the body's energy field. Intuitives in our culture can see this energy field as light or colors emanating from the body. When a person is calm, relaxed, and healthy, the energy field appears radiant and full of colors. The colors tend to be bright and harmonious. When we are feeling anxious or tense, we lose light and color. Our energy field looks more discordant and jagged, and often the colors change to duller, more muddied colors. Color breathing is a technique that can help strengthen and heal the energy field as well as calm the mind and body. As you breathe in the healing colors, you often begin to relax and feel healthier again. Anxiety and tension are replaced by a sensation of lightness and peace.

- Sit or lie in a comfortable position.

- Imagine a cloud of beautiful golden energy surrounding you. As you take a deep breath, inhale the golden energy and visualize it flowing through your body—a healing energy that warms and relaxes you.

- Hold the inhalation as long as it is comfortable. Let this golden cloud pick up all your anxiety and tension.

- Then, exhale this energy out through your lungs and let it be carried away from you.

- Repeat this process as many times as needed until a feeling of peace and calm replaces your anxiety.

Exercise 5: Emotional Healing Breath

I have seen, during my years of medical practice, that negative feelings and belief systems are major triggers of anxiety, nervous tension, and even physical illness. This exercise again uses color breathing to help you release negative feelings such as chronic anger, hurt, or other upsets you may be harboring. The more time you spend cleansing old negative emotional patterns, the less impact they will have on your moods and your life.

- Lie flat on your back with your knees pulled up. Keep your feet slightly apart. Try to breathe in and out through your nose.

- Inhale deeply and see yourself enveloped in a soft white light. Breathe this light into every cell of your body. This is a cleansing light and can help wash away fear, anger, anxiety, and other negative feelings.

- As you exhale, feel the light washing these emotions away.

- Repeat this exercise until you feel emotionally peaceful and clear.

Exercise 6: Muscle-Tension Release Breathing

This exercise will help you to get in touch with and release general muscle tension and tightness. Often when we are anxious and upset, we unconsciously tense up muscles throughout the entire body. The neck, shoulders, lower back, and other areas of the body are particularly vulnerable. This exercise will help you focus on any tension that you are carrying in your upper body. Relaxing and releasing the muscles in your neck and shoulders will help release muscle tension in your entire body. To get in touch with any muscle tension that you may be carrying, use this exercise while walking or doing sports or desk work.

- Sit upright in a chair. Be sure you are in a comfortable position. Keep your feet slightly apart. Try to breathe in and out through your nose.

- Inhale and exhale deeply. As you breathe, let your head move from side to side. Keep your shoulders down and try to touch your ear to your shoulder. As you do this movement, imagine that your neck is made out of putty and that it allows your head to move in a supple, relaxed movement from the left to the right.

- Now inhale and pull your shoulders up towards your ears. Hold your breath and keep your shoulders in a hunched position. Exhale and let your shoulders drop back into a relaxed, comfortable position. Repeat this several times.

- Inhale and exhale deeply as you roll your shoulders forward. Make a large, slow, circular motion with your shoulders. Then roll your shoulders back slowly, again inhaling and exhaling. Repeat this sequence several times.

- Inhale and exhale deeply, keeping the rest of your body still and relaxed. Repeat this several times.

Exercise 7: Glandular Breathing

Anxiety and nervous tension often deplete endocrine gland function. Women with depleted endocrine glands may not only feel stressed and tired, but may also be prone to imbalances like PMS, menopause symptoms, hypoglycemia, and hyperthyroidism. In addition, they may also be more likely to develop infections like colds and flu, because the endocrine glands help regulate the immune function.

This exercise helps stimulate and energize your endocrine glands through the use of color breathing. When you direct your breath into the endocrine glands and visualize them being stimulated by the color, the glands are, in fact, stimulated in a beneficial way. The use of color breathing expands the glands' electromagnetic field. In this exercise, the color red is used; in research studies, red light has been shown to stimulate both the endocrine and immune functions.

- Sit upright in a chair, your arms at your sides, palms up. Imagine a large balloon filled with the color red above your head. It is a bright, vibrant tone of red that sparkles with energy. As you inhale deeply, see yourself popping this balloon and releasing the color red. See the color red flowing into your head and concentrating in the hypothalamus, a gland located at the base of the brain. As the hypothalamus begins to overflow with color, exhale and breathe the red out of your lungs, filling the air around you.

- As you inhale again, breathe the bright red color into your pituitary, an important endocrine gland located in your brain, right below the hypothalamus. Fill the pituitary with this color until it overflows. Then exhale deeply.

- As you continue to inhale the bright red color, let it flow into your thyroid gland, located in your neck, then into your thymus gland, located in the middle of your chest. Finally, let the color energize your adrenal glands, located in the middle of your back above the kidneys, and your ovaries, located in the pelvis. When you finish this exercise, relax for a few minutes.

Exercise 8: Depression Release Breathing

Depression and fatigue often accompany anxiety in women with mood swings. It is very upsetting to swing between feeling anxious and irritable on the one hand and feeling blue and down on the other; there is never a sense of proper emotional balance. Such mood swings may have psychological origins or may result from PMS, menopause, and hypoglycemia. This next exercise helps elevate mood and enhance emotional well-being through focused breathing.

- Sit upright in a chair. Cross your arms in front of your chest with your fingers touching the upper outer area of your chest. Your wrist crosses over your heart chakra, which is the energy center for emotions and feelings in traditional Oriental healing models.

- As you inhale, imagine a golden light filling your heart center with a warm, loving feeling. As you exhale, breathe out depression and low spirits.

- As you inhale again, draw this golden light up through your neck and into your head. See it illuminating your head with a soft, peaceful glow. Feel any depression or negative thoughts dissolving as the golden light fills every cell in your brain.

- As you exhale, breathe the golden light out through the top of your head and see it form a shimmering cloud of energy around your entire body.

- Repeat the exercise five times.

Putting Your Breathing Exercise Program Together

This chapter suggests many effective exercises to help reduce anxiety and tension through controlled breathing. Try each exercise once and choose those that you enjoy the most to practice on a regular basis. These exercises can help you even if you practice them only a few minutes each day. Over time, healthy breathing habits will become automatic and will greatly benefit your general health.

8

Physical Exercises

Exercise is an important part of your anxiety and stress reduction program. The discharge of physical and emotional tension that accompanies a vigorous session of exercise directly and immediately reduces anxiety and stress. In addition, the long-term physiological benefits of exercise build up your resistance to stress and promote beneficial psychological changes. Let us look at how exercise produces these changes in the body and mind.

The Benefits of Exercise

Exercise Improves Resistance to and Relief of Anxiety Episodes

When women have excessive anxiety and tension due to lifestyle stress or emotional problems, the sympathetic nervous system is easily tripped, producing the fight-or-flight response. The same is true for women who are in a state of hormonal or physiological imbalance caused by PMS, menopause, hypoglycemia, overactivity of the thyroid, or mitral valve prolapse.

The problem for many women who have chronic anxiety and tension is that their sympathetic nervous system is always in a state of readiness to a crisis. This puts them in a constant state of tension, causing them to react to small stresses the same way they react to real emergencies. Their adrenal glands increase their output of adrenaline and cortisone, and their thyroid gland pumps out thyroxin (the thyroid hormone), adjusting the body chemistry to meet the crisis. Their heart speeds up, their pulses race, and their neck and shoulder muscles tense, as do muscles in other parts of the body.

These tight and tense muscles have decreased blood flow and oxygenation. Waste products such as excessive carbon dioxide accumulate in this physical environment and can further worsen fight-or-flight symptoms. In addition, stress causes breathing to become rapid and shallow. Less oxygen is taken in through respiration, which further decreases the oxygen available to the muscles and internal organs.

The tension that accumulates in the body to meet this "emergency" must then be discharged. Often it is discharged emotionally by yelling at children or being rude and abrupt with people at work. Some women deal with this fight-or-flight reaction by discharging their anxiety through harmful food, alcohol, or cigarette addictions. For example, overeating becomes a way of diffusing tension. The habitual indulgence in addictive behavior is additionally harmful to the body.

Physical exercise, particularly aerobic types, discharges the fight-or-flight tension without harming either your personal relationships or your body. Exercise improves oxygenation and blood circulation to tight muscles and devitalized organ systems. By improving circulation, exercise facilitates proper nutrient flow throughout the body. Removal of waste products such as carbon dioxide, lactic acid, and other products of metabolism becomes more efficient. The acidity or pH of the blood is lowered to an optimal range, and the production of energy by the cells becomes more efficient. This is important since optimal energy production is needed to run the body's many chemical and physiological functions.

With regular exercise, skeletal muscles become energized and toned, making every movement—from lifting objects to walking—more easily accomplished. The heart muscle also works more efficiently. As the heart becomes conditioned, it is able to pump more blood with each stroke. Thus, it can circulate the same volume of blood with fewer strokes and doesn't have to work as hard. Once an exercise program is initiated, the resting heart rate soon slows down quite markedly. Research studies show that the beneficial changes can occur rapidly, often within several months.

A lower resting heart rate means more than increased strength and stamina. A healthier heart also reacts less dramatically during episodes of anxiety and stress. When anxiety causes the adrenal glands to pump out stressor hormones, a conditioned heart will not experience a significant rise in the heart rate. In a stressful situation, a fit person may have only a slight rise in heart rate, while a sedentary person may experience a terrifying pounding of the heart and shortness of breath. Not only does a fit woman tend to stay calmer and more in control of her emotions during a taxing situation, but also in periods of extreme stress, her good physical conditioning may help prevent a heart attack and thereby save her life.

Exercise Improves Brain Function

Besides improving cardiovascular function, regular exercise also reduces anxiety by improving brain function. Healthy brain function is necessary to decrease nervous tension and reduce the tendency toward panic episodes and phobias. After exercising, you will feel more peaceful, calmer, and even happier. You will certainly feel more refreshed and energized. How does exercise promote such striking emotional changes? Exercise brings better oxygenation and circulation to the brain and nerves by opening up and dilating blood vessels of the head and brain. Thus, more nutrients can flow into and more waste products can be removed from this vital system. In fact, 20 percent of the blood flow from the heart goes directly to the brain. The brain also utilizes a large share (again, 20 percent) of the body's nutrients and energy.

Research studies done on adults who exercise compared with similar groups who are sedentary show striking differences in a variety of mental functions. Adults engaged in an active exercise program have better concentration, and clearer and quicker thinking and problem solving. In addition, reaction time and short-term memory improve.

Not only does regular exercise induce functional improvements in the brain, it also dramatically alters brain chemistry in a positive way through the increased production of beta endorphins. Beta endorphins, chemicals released from the pituitary glands, act as natural opiates. They are chemically similar to the pain reliever morphine, but 200 times more potent. Endorphins have a dramatic effect on mood. When levels in the body are high, they improve a woman's general sense of well-being. Beta endorphin levels increase after ovulation, during the early part of the second half of the menstrual cycle (called the luteal phase by physicians). As menstruation approaches, beta endorphin levels can begin to fall. In fact, some PMS researchers believe that the drop in beta endorphins may be responsible for the emotional symptoms of PMS such as anxiety, irritability, and mood swings. These are the predominant symptoms in more than 80 percent of women with PMS.

Exercise helps reduce anxiety and nervous tension by increasing the production of beta endorphins. Research studies demonstrate that brisk aerobic exercise like running can increase beta endorphin levels as much as fivefold. Measurements of beta endorphins taken a half hour after the exercise session showed that beta endorphin levels were still higher than at starting. In fact, beta endorphins are thought to be responsible for the "runner's high" that marathoners experience. Some women who exercise regularly report related feelings of elation, euphoria, and even bliss. Aerobic exercise may even help cushion the premenstrual fall in beta endorphins and thereby reduce PMS-related anxiety.

Exercise Improves Psychological Function

Since the beta endorphins tend to elevate mood and promote well-being, exercise can also be an effective antidote for depression. While the standard treatment for depression is psychotherapy and antidepressant medication, a number of interesting chemical studies have shown that exercise significantly helps relieve moderate depression. One interesting study, done at the University of Virginia, observed depressed college students. Those who jogged regularly during the period of the study showed significant reduction in depression symptoms, while those who did not exercise during the same period had virtually no change in their symptoms. This finding has significance for women who suffer from anxiety and nervous tension, since anxiety and depression often occur together. Psychotherapists who treat women for emotional disorders are aware that these two conditions frequently coexist. Even with health issues like PMS and menopause, which are primarily due to a variety of hormonal and chemical imbalances (rather than emotional causes), anxiety and depression frequently coexist. Women with these problems will complain that their mood vacillates between nervous or irritable and depressed. Exercise can be a powerful antidote for problems on both ends of the emotional spectrum.

Women who are anxious and nervous often have difficulty sleeping at night. They may lie in bed for two to three hours, their minds busy with "chatter" and self-talk. Often this self-talk includes fearful thoughts and worries about stressful life situations or even imagined concerns. Some women have difficulty sleeping when their anxiety is mixed with strong anger, hostility, and upset toward a person or difficult situation. I have had anxious patients tell me that they have tried strong sleeping medications or alcoholic beverages to induce sleep; however, upset feelings can override the sedative effects of the medication or alcohol. This can lead to drug and alcohol abuse as women increase their intake in an effort to shut off their disturbing thoughts and feelings at night.

Exercise can help to reduce insomnia by working off nervous energy and diffusing the fight-or-flight response. After exercise, both the body and mind are calmer. It is often easier for women to relax and sleep soundly when they have included a session of physical activity in their daily schedule. Exercise should not, however, be done late in the day by women suffering from insomnia, since the energizing effects of the exercise are not desirable late at night. It is better to exercise earlier in the day if sleep induction is one of your main goals.

Other psychological benefits can come from the act of exercising itself. Regular exercise demands discipline and a willingness to overcome resistance and inertia. Anxious and stressed women often feel as if their life is out of control or their life's structure is falling apart. This is particularly true for women who have frequent panic attacks, are crippled by phobias, or suffer from a constant high level of anxiety and nervousness. Choosing specific times to exercise and then exercising on a regular basis provides structure and discipline. A woman who begins a session of running, brisk walking, or golf feeling anxious will often find her mind focusing on the activity itself or the attractive surroundings, such as a golf course or swimming area. As the session progresses, tension will fade away. Also, since many forms of exercise or sport do require a level of skill mastery, regular physical activity gives a tremendous boost of self-confidence in women who feel they have no control over their emotions. Mastery of a physical skill provides the blueprint for handling emotional upsets more effectively. This allows you to deal with your problems with more self-esteem, an improved self-image, and greater coping skills.

Many people also perceive exercise as a good habit. Often women consciously substitute exercise for more harmful ways that they have dealt with stress in the past, such as overeating, alcohol abuse, or combative behavior. Exercising regularly, three to five times a week, is a positive "addiction" that has many beneficial effects on health.

Exercise Improves Physiological Functions

Exercise can also have a beneficial effect on anxiety due to physiological factors. For instance, exercise helps to reduce stress symptoms due to hypoglycemia or PMS-related sugar cravings by stabilizing the blood sugar level. Along with diet, exercise can help reduce the tendency toward such common hypoglycemia symptoms as anxiety, jitteriness, inability to concentrate, and dizziness. Exercise helps iron out the roller coaster blood sugar highs and lows from which women with hypoglycemia suffer.

Exercise has a benefical effect on our intake and processing of food. First, it reduces excessive cravings for food, both for women with food addictions and for women with PMS who tend to overeat high-stress foods in the week or two prior to the onset of menstruation. This curbing of excessive appetite and overeating improves our ability to lose and maintain weight. Second, exercise inproves the body's ability to burn calories more efficiently and rapidly. This provides an additional boost to weight loss.

Exercise benefits the general health of many other systems, too. Elimination through the bowels and kidneys is improved, which also helps to regulate weight and water balance. Constipation is less likely to be a problem in active women. It reduces the tendency to anxiety-related digestive symptoms such as abdominal discomfort and bloating. In fact, I have had patients with stress-related intestinal symptoms report symptom relief immediately following exercise sessions. Exercise also helps reduce blood pressure levels, which takes stress off the heart and contributes to a reduction of heart attack risk. In summary, exercise benefits the entire body and promotes good health.

Benefits of Exercise

Improves resistance to and relief of anxiety episodes
- Reduces the fight-or-flight response
- Promotes cardiovascular resistance to stress
- Decreases skeletal muscle tension
- Reduces pent-up aggression and frustration
- Promotes a feeling of calm and peace

Improves brain function
- Promotes better oxygenation and blood circulation to the brain
- Increases output of beta endorphins
- Improves concentration, problem solving, reaction time, and short-term memory

Improves psychological functions
- Decreases anxiety and nervous tension
- Produces a sense of well-being and even elation
- Reduces depression
- Reduces insomnia
- Improves sense of mastery and self-confidence
- Promotes development of beneficial habits
- Helps decrease harmful addictive behavior

Improves physiological functions
- Stabilizes blood sugar level
- Reduces food craving
- Helps weight loss and maintenance
- Improves elimination through the bowels and kidneys
- Improves digestive functions
- Reduces blood pressure

Building Your Exercise Program

Evaluating Your Fitness Level

If you are currently making the transition from a sedentary life-style to a regular exercise program, evaluate your level of fitness. It is important to know if you have any undiagnosed medical problems that could affect your proper level of activity. These would include problems like thyroid disease and hypoglycemia, which can trigger anxiety symptoms in connection with exercise. I have had patients with thyroid imbalance, for example, who felt more anxious and short of breath when exercising, because their excessive levels of thyroid hormone were elevating their heart and pulse rates to unhealthy levels during times of increased activity.

If you have not already done so, I recommend that you fill out the workbook section questionnaires on your current exercise habits, patterns of muscle tension, and symptoms of lack of physical fitness. If you find you have chronic muscle tension or feel out-of-breath after walking up a flight of stairs, you may actually have an underlying problem like anemia (low red blood cell count), which can often go undiagnosed if the symptoms are merely imputed to a sedentary lifestyle. In fact, I suggest that you share your responses to these questionnaires with your health-care provider because they may offer valuable clues to help discover a medical problem that hasn't yet been diagnosed. Be sure to let your physician know if you have any previously diagnosed problems such as mitral valve prolapse, which can also trigger anxiety-like episodes.

Your physician should check your heart, lungs, pulse rate, and other physical parameters to evaluate your exercise fitness. In addition, blood and urine tests are frequently ordered. These tests can vary based on the particular symptoms you describe to your physician as well as on the examination itself. Depending on the age of the woman, blood sugar, thyroid, and menopause blood tests are frequently used when screening for anxiety. If you don't understand any terms or tests used, ask your physician for more information. An informed and educated woman patient can do a much better job planning and participating in her own wellness program. Once you have received a clean bill of health or understand any health limitations, you are ready to begin planning your exercise program.

Choosing an Exercise Program

The type of exercise regimen you choose can vary greatly depending on the goals you wish to accomplish. If your main goal is to relieve anxiety and stress and improve your general health and well-being, then aerobic exercise is best. Aerobic exercise includes jogging, walking, bicycle riding, skiing, swimming, dancing, jumping rope, and skating. Aerobic exercise reduces stress, promotes calm and relaxation, and helps reduce the tendency toward insomnia and addictive food and drug behavior. Because it requires active work on the part of your skeletal and heart muscles, it reduces the muscle tension that often accompanies anxiety and improves cardiovascular fitness, oxygenation, and circulation to all the systems of the body, thereby increasing your resistance to stress.

If you need to discharge pent-up anger and frustration, competitive sports such as handball, squash, racquetball, tennis, and soccer may be best, so you can work out your aggressions in fast-paced and demanding competitive play. If you find that simply socializing and playing games with other people helps to reduce nervous tension and stress, then slower-paced sports and games like golf, croquet, and bowling could provide such relaxation.

For those women whose anxiety and stress symptoms include significant muscle tightness and tension, exercises that promote muscular flexibility, like yoga and other stretching exercises, can be very helpful. Yoga stretches are performed slowly, along with deep breathing, in a relaxed and careful manner. They are helpful in slowing down an anxious system whose physiology is set on overdrive.

Types of Exercise

- Jogging
- Walking
- Bicycle riding
- Skiing
- Swimming
- Aerobic dancing
- Jumping rope
- Ice skating
- Roller skating
- Handball
- Racquetball
- Squash
- Tennis
- Soccer
- Basketball
- Baseball
- Table tennis
- Golf
- Croquet
- Bowling
- Yoga
- Stretching
- Weight lifting
- Gardening

If increased muscle strength and definition are important for your self-image as well as increasing stamina, then weight lifting can be an important part of your exercise regimen. Finally, if being outdoors while you discharge anxiety and tension works for you, gardening can be very healing. Bending, lifting, and upper-body movements dissipate anxiety and upset rapidly while you are pulling weeds and digging up the ground for new plantings.

Often, women may combine two or three types of exercise activities to meet a variety of goals. Whatever form of exercise you choose, make sure that it meets the goals of reducing anxiety and stress and promoting an improved sense of calm and well-being.

Keeping an Exercise Diary

Keep an exercise diary during the first few months of a new exercise program. I have included a diary form in the workbook section that you can use. You will derive many benefits by keeping an exercise diary. Women subject to anxiety episodes, panic attacks, and phobias often feel out of control. When experiencing an anxiety episode, it is difficult to organize and carry through with your activities. This can hamper effective performance in many different areas of life, not just exercise. The use of an exercise diary provides the helpful organizational guide that you need to initiate, carry out, and then evaluate the exercise program that you have chosen. This will enable you to determine if your program is providing you with the maximum anxiety-reducing benefits.

When filling out the diary, record the dates on which you exercised, the type of exercise you engaged in, and your emotional and physical responses to the exercise session. If you skipped a planned session, be sure to record the reason why, such as illness or excessive work demands. Record both positive and negative responses to your exercise session. When recording your emotional responses, be sure to note if your anxiety, panic, or stress symptoms actually increase. This can occur if you are pushing

Optimal Pulse Ranges by Age

Age	Pulse Rate (also indicates heart rate)
20–29	145–164
30–39	138–156
40–49	130–148
50–59	122–140
60–69+	116–132

yourself too hard with an exercise program that is too vigorous or demanding. In this case, you may want to reduce the length of time you are exercising, the intensity with which you exercise, or the type of physical activity you're doing.

In monitoring your physical responses to exercise, choose such parameters as beneficial changes in muscle tension and pulse rate. When doing aerobic exercise, your pulse rate should measure in the optimal range for your age. (See the table in the margin for the pulse ranges for various age groups.)

Do not continue with an exercise program if it doesn't meet your ultimate goal: reduction of anxiety, stress, and their associated symptoms. With such a wide range of exercises and sports to choose from, you can use your diary to help you determine what mix of physical activities works best for you.

Motivating Yourself to Exercise

If you encounter mental obstacles to beginning and sticking with a regular exercise program, there are many ways to overcome this resistance. Be sure that you are clear why you don't want to exercise so that you can address the issues directly. Keeping the exercise diary found in the workbook section should help you pinpoint areas of resistance.

- Make sure you exercise at the time of day that feels most natural. For example, if you are a late riser, don't try to exercise early in the morning. Exercise when you are the least hurried and stressed by your schedule. If your largest amount of free time is in the late afternoon between work and dinner, put aside that time to engage in physical activity.

- Exercise in an attractive setting. If you run or walk, pick a setting near you that promotes peace and calm. Walk or run in a park, beach, or even a quiet residential street. Avoid areas with lots of cars and traffic congestion.

- Exercise with a friend or support person. This can be a great help in motivating and encouraging you to begin and stick with an exercise program.

- Use your mind to disconnect from your daily activities. Positive mental exercises can help you to relax before starting physical activity. Many women find that a few minutes of doing visualizations (seeing themselves performing and enjoying the exercise routine in their minds) or saying affirmations (positive statements about the benefits of exercise) prepares them for their exercise routine.

- Listen to music while you exercise. Many women find that the exercise period goes by much more quickly and the process is more fun and enjoyable when they listen to music. Be sure to choose music that is mellow and relaxing since it will help improve your mood and relax you further.

- Be sure to choose an exercise activity that you enjoy. Don't pick an activity that worsens your anxiety level or that you find boring. Refer to the chart of Types of Exercise in this chapter if you need help in selecting an activity that is fun and interesting for you.

Beginning an Exercise Program for Relief of Anxiety and Stress

Before you begin your exercise program for relief of anxiety and stress, read through the following guidelines. They will help you to perform your exercise program in an optimal manner. These guidelines are particularly good for women who are just beginning an exercise program after leading a sedentary life. They are also helpful for women who have previously been fit and active but stopped exercising because physical exertion seemed to trigger anxiety, panic episodes, or muscle tension. An exercise program that is too strenuous can leave a woman with anxiety feeling more anxious and uptight than ever. Thus, getting a good start on an exercise program can make a major difference in how well you can stick to and even enjoy your chosen physical activity.

- During the first week or two of your program, build up your exercise level gradually. Limit your initial exercise workouts to short sessions. For example, you might start out exercising every other day for only 10 minutes. Then, increase the length of your sessions gradually in 5-minute increments until you are exercising between 30 and 60 minutes per session.

- Perform the exercise in a relaxed and unhurried manner. Be sure to set aside adequate time so you do not feel rushed. Anytime you feel anxiety, panic, or excessive muscle tension, stop doing the exercise. Then re-evaluate your pace to see if it is too vigorous. Initially you might want to exercise with another person who can provide support if your anxiety symptoms become very severe.

- Wear loose, comfortable clothing. If you are doing stretching or yoga, work without socks to give your feet complete freedom of movement and to prevent slipping.

- Evacuate your bowels or bladder before you begin the exercises. Try to exercise at least 90 minutes before a meal and wait at least two hours after eating to exercise. Working out before dinner is particularly good since it helps diffuse tensions that have accumulated throughout the day.

- Avoid exercising when you are ill or during times of extreme stress. At such times, the stress-reduction exercises or breathing exercises provided in this book will be more useful.

- Move slowly and carefully when first starting to exercise. This will help promote flexibility of the muscles and prevent injury.

- Always rest for a few minutes after finishing a session.

9

Yoga for Relief of Anxiety & Stress

Yoga stretches provide effective relief of anxiety and stress. Always perform them slowly and carefully and accompany the stretches with deep, relaxed breathing. Yoga stretches quiet your mood and promote a deep sense of peace and calm. Unlike fast-paced aerobic exercise, yoga actually slows down your pulse, heart rate, and breathing. This benefits many women with anxiety and tension related to life stress. Yoga provides an oasis of calm in which you can put aside your stress and focus on doing the exercises slowly and on breathing calmly and deeply.

When you practice a series of yoga exercises, you gently stretch every muscle in your body. These exercises relax tense muscles and improve their suppleness and flexibility. They also promote better circulation and oxygenation to tense and contracted areas throughout the body. As a result, general metabolism of the muscles and organ system is improved. Both the stress reduction effects and the physiological effects of yoga benefit all body systems, including digestive and elimination function, the endocrine (glandular) system, the nervous system, and the immune system.

I have included in this chapter a series of yoga poses that specifically reduce anxiety and stress. Some of these exercises work on the emotions, calming your mood and inducing peace and serenity. Other poses help relieve the physical causes of anxiety and stress, such as PMS and menopause-related problems.

I recommend reading through the exercises first to see which ones apply to your causes of anxiety and stress. You may want to try these exercises first. Or you could try all the exercises initially for the first week or two and see which ones produce the most beneficial results. You can do the yoga stretches three times a week, or even daily if your anxiety and stress symptoms respond well to more frequent practice.

When you begin the anxiety and stress-relief exercises, it is important that you focus your mind and concentrate on the positions. First your mind visualizes how the exercise is to look, then your body follows with the correct execution of the pose. Pay close attention to the initial instructions. Look carefully at the placement of the body in the photographs. If you practice the stretch properly, you are much more likely to have relief of your symptoms.

Move through each pose slowly. This slowness allows you to have greater control over your body movements. You minimize the possibility of injury and maximize the benefit to the particular part of the body that is the focus of the pose. If you practice these yoga stretches regularly in an unhurried fashion, you will also gradually loosen your muscles, ligaments, and joints. You may be surprised at how supple you can become.

If you experience any pain or discomfort, you have probably overreached your current ability and should immediately reduce the amount of the stretching until you can proceed without discomfort. Be careful, as muscular injuries can take quite awhile to heal. If you do strain a muscle, apply ice to the injured area for 10 minutes. Use the ice pack two to three times a day for several days. If the pain persists, see your doctor.

Follow the breathing instructions for the exercise. Most important, do not hold your breath. Allow your breath to flow in and out easily and effortlessly.

Stretch 1: Child's Pose

This exercise is excellent for calming anxiety and stress due to emotional causes, and it will also relieve anxiety and irritability due to PMS and menopause. For women with food addiction episodes or coexisting mitral valve prolapse, it will lessen anxiety. This exercise gently stretches the lower back and is one of the most effective exercises for relieving menstrual cramps.

- Sit on your heels. Bring your forehead to the floor, stretching the spine as far as possible.

- Close your eyes.

- Hold for as long as comfortable.

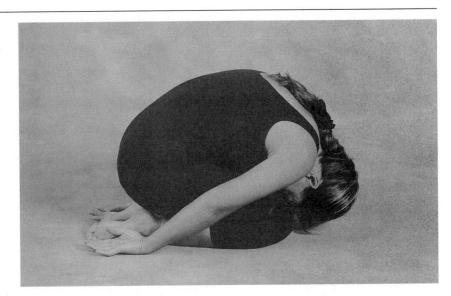

Stretch 2: The Sponge

This exercise relieves anxiety and stress due to emotional causes, PMS, or menopause. It helps quiet anxiety in women with coexisting food addiction episodes or mitral valve prolapse. It relieves menstrual cramps and low back pain. It also reduces eye tension and swelling in the face.

- Lie on your back with a rolled towel placed under your knees. Your arms should be at your sides, palms up.

- Close your eyes and relax your whole body. Inhale slowly, breathing from the diaphragm. As you inhale, visualize the energy in the air around you being drawn in through your entire body. Imagine that your body is porous and open like a sponge, so it can draw in this energy to revitalize every cell of your body.

- Exhale slowly and deeply, allowing every ounce of tension to drain from your body.

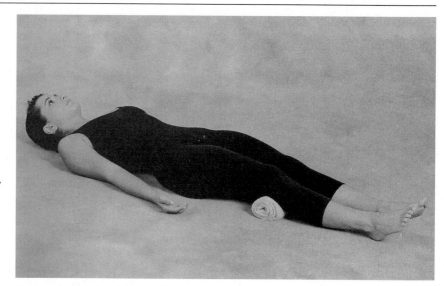

Stretch 3: Rock and Roll

This exercise massages the neck and spine and flexes the vertebral column. It will invigorate and energize you, helping balance your body and mind and reduce fatigue. It also promotes good circulation and relieves low back tension. To enhance the benefits of the exercise, lie flat on your back for a few minutes after doing it.

- Lie on your back. Bend and raise your knees to your chest, clasping them with your hands. Hands should be interlocked below and in front of knees.

- Raise your head toward your knees and gently rock back and forth on your curved spine. Note the roundness of your back and shoulders. Inhale slowly as you come up and exhale slowly as you go back. Keep your chin tucked in as you roll back. Avoid rolling back too far on your neck.

- Rock back and forth 5 to 10 times.

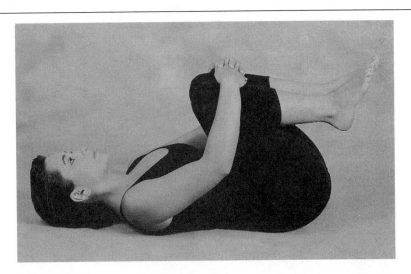

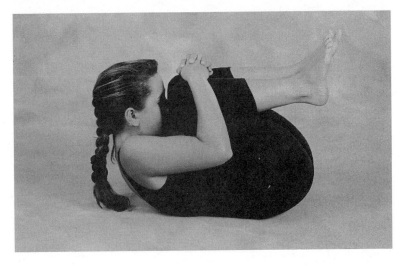

Stretch 4: Dollar Pose

This pose reduces anxiety and nervous tension and will help eliminate tension headaches and insomnia. It improves flexibility of the spine, reducing stiffness and back pain.

- Lie on your back with your legs bent and your feet together. Place your hands on the sides of both ankles to keep your legs together.

- As you inhale, raise your legs up over your head. To make sure that the posture is comfortable, adjust the angle of your legs, bending your knees to apply pressure between the shoulder blades.

- Hold this posture for one minute, breathing slowly and deeply.

- Return to the original position, lying flat on your back with your eyes closed. Relax in this position for several minutes.

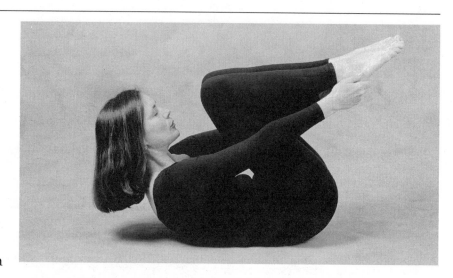

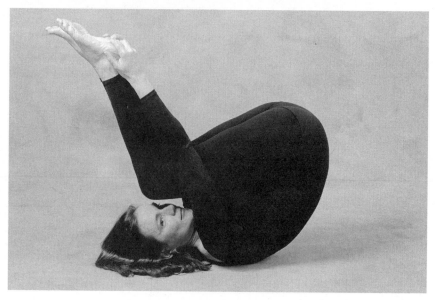

Stretch 5: The Pump

This exercise calms anxiety and nervousness. It strengthens the back and abdominal muscles and improves blood circulation and oxygenation to the pelvis.

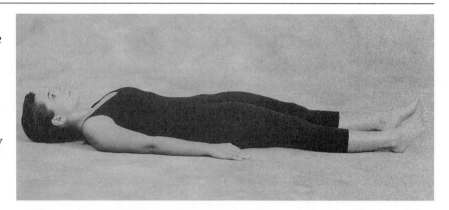

- Lie down and press the small of your back into the floor. This permits you to use your abdominal muscles without straining your lower back.

- Raise your right leg slowly while breathing in. Keep your back flat on the floor and let the rest of your body remain relaxed. Move your leg very slowly; imagine your leg being lifted up smoothly by a pulley. Do not move your leg in a jerking manner. Hold for a few breaths.

- Lower your leg and breathe out.

- Repeat the same exercise on your left side. Then alternate legs, repeating the exercise 5 to 10 times.

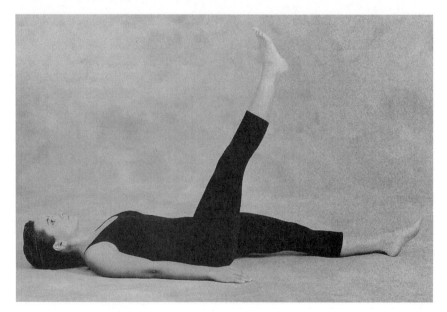

Stretch 6: Cobra Pose

This exercise reduces anxiety and nervous tension. It also helps to eliminate tension headaches. By stretching the spine, you enhance circulation and improve spinal flexibility.

- Lie on your stomach with your chin on the floor and your feet together. Place your palms flat on the floor, underneath your shoulders.

- As you inhale, lift your head up, stretching your neck back. Then, raise your chest, using your arms and back muscles.

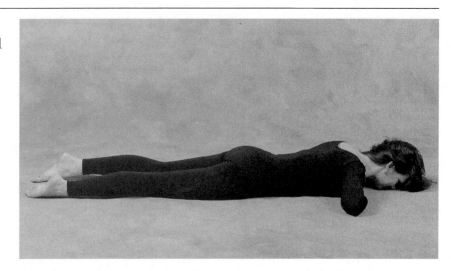

- As you complete the inhalation, arch your body all the way up, keeping your hips on the ground.

- As you hold this position, exhale deeply. Then, breathe deeply and slowly, inhaling and exhaling for 30 seconds.

- Lower yourself part way, using your arms for support. Holding the body at this angle, breathe deeply for 30 seconds.

- Then let your body come all the way down. Relax with your head turned to one side and your arms resting gently on the floor. Close your eyes and relax for several minutes.

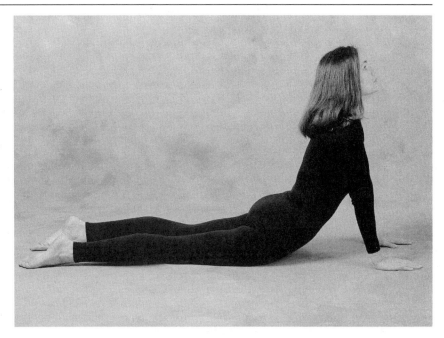

Stretch 7: Boat Pose

This exercise helps release overall body tension. It improves circulation and concentration. It strengthens the lower back and abdominal area.

• Lie on your stomach with your feet together and your arms lying flat at your sides.

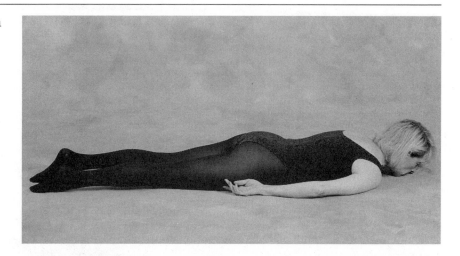

• Stretch your arms out straight in front of you on the floor.

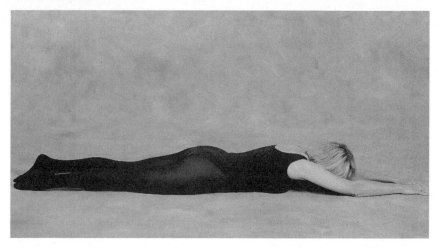

- As you inhale, arch your back and lift your arms, head, chest and legs off the floor. Hold the pose as long as you can, up to 30 seconds, breathing deeply and slowly.

- Return to the original resting position with your head turned to the side, and completely relax for 1 to 3 minutes.

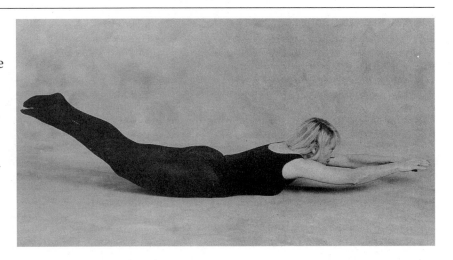

Stretch 8: Side Rolls

This exercise helps relieve emotional tension and frustration. By helping release emotional upset locked in the muscles, this stretch promotes a sense of relaxation, mental balance, improved energy, and vitality.

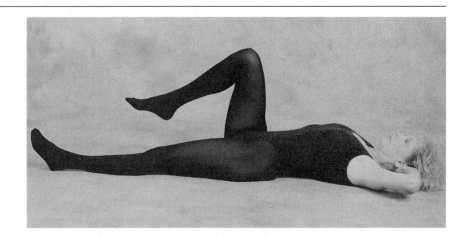

- Lie on your back with your hands interlaced under your neck.

- As you inhale, bend and lift your right leg.

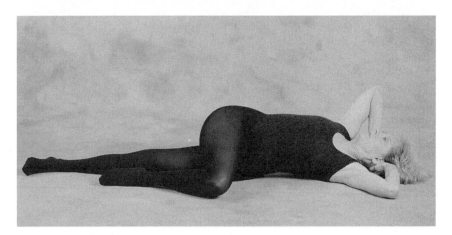

- Then exhale and roll on your left side, with your left knee touching the ground. As you do this, release a sigh.

- As you inhale, return to your original position.

- Repeat this 10 times, alternating sides.

- Then relax on your back for 1 minute.

Stretch 9: The Locust

This exercise helps relieve PMS- and menopause-related anxiety and stress and other premenstrual and menopausal symptoms by energizing the female reproductive tract. It also energizes the liver, intestines, and kidneys, and strengthens the lower back, abdomen, buttocks, and legs.

- Lie face down on the floor. Make fists with both your hands and place them under your hips. This prevents compression of the lumbar spine while doing the exercise.

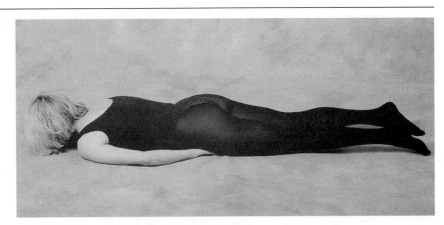

- Straighten your body and raise your right leg with an upward thrust as high as you can, keeping your hips on your fists. Hold for 5 to 20 seconds if possible.

- Lower the leg and slowly return to your original position. Repeat with the left leg, then with both legs together. Remember to keep your hips resting on your fists.

- Repeat 10 times.

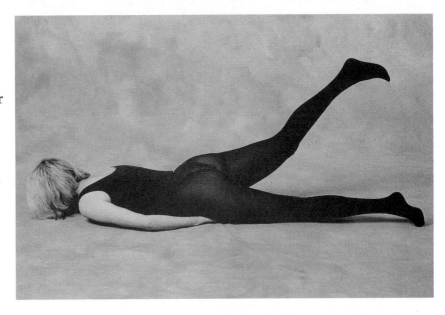

Stretch 10: The Bow

This exercise is one of the most powerful stretches for increasing total body energy and vitality and releasing muscle tension. It strengthens the nervous system, balances the mood, may reduce sugar craving, and helps reduce anxiety and nervous tension. It improves concentration and mental clarity. It also stimulates the thyroid, thymus, liver, kidneys, and female reproductive tract, and improves digestive function.

- Lie face down on the floor, arms at your sides.

- Slowly bend your legs at the knees and bring your feet up toward your buttocks.

- Reach back with your arms and carefully take hold of first one foot and then the other. Flex your feet to make grasping them easier.

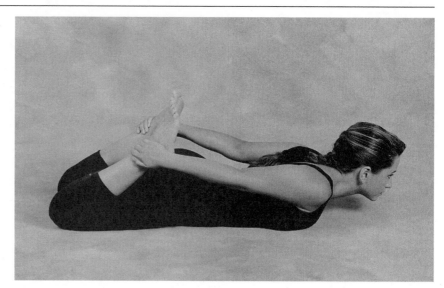

- As you inhale, lift your head and raise your trunk from the floor as far as possible. Bring your knees together and lift your legs off the floor as far as possible, too. Imagine your body looking like a gently curved bow. Hold for 10 to 15 seconds.

- Slowly release the posture. Allow your chin to touch the floor and finally release your feet and return them slowly to the floor. Return to your original position.

- Repeat 5 times.

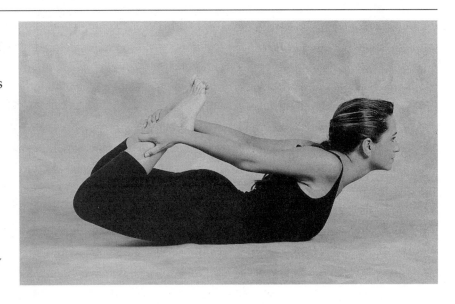

Stretch 11: Half-Wheel Pose

This exercise helps relieve nervous tension and stress, tension headaches, and menstrual problems. It also helps prevent colds and respiratory infections. Use it to relieve allergic and respiratory symptoms.

• Lie on your back with your knees bent and the bottoms of your feet flat on the floor.

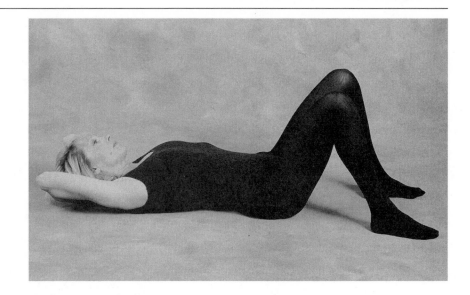

- Bring your hands under your neck with the backs of your hands pressing against each other and the knuckles of your smallest fingers pressing into the base of your skull. Spread your index finger and thumb apart on each hand.

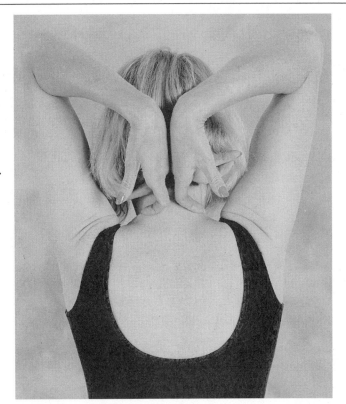

- Inhale deeply and arch your hips up. Breathe deeply in this position for up to 1 minute.

- As you exhale, slowly come down and return to your original position.

- Relax in this position for 1 to 3 minutes.

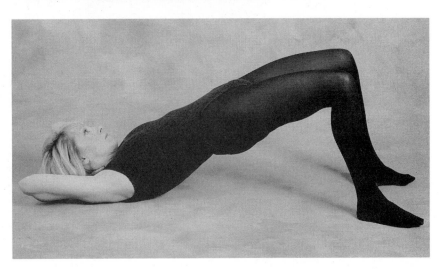

10

Acupressure for Relief of Anxiety & Stress

Acupressure helps relieve both the emotional and the physical causes of anxiety and stress. Based on an ancient Oriental healing technique, it involves applying gentle finger pressure to specific points on the skin. Unlike acupuncture, which requires the use of needles and many years of training, acupressure can be easily learned and performed.

I have recommended the use of simple acupressure points to my patients for many years, and I have been pleased with the positive feedback they give me. Many of them have told me that they feel calmer and more peaceful after working with acupressure. This chapter includes easy-to-follow directions and many photographs of specific exercises, which should make acupressure easy for you.

About Acupressure

Pressing specific acupressure points creates changes on two levels. On the physical level, acupressure affects muscular tension, blood circulation, and other physiological parameters. On a more subtle level, according to traditional Oriental medicine, acupressure also builds the body's life energy, thereby promoting healing. In fact, acupressure is based on the belief that the body contains a life energy called *chi.* It is different from, yet similar to, electromagnetic energy. Health can be viewed as a state in which the chi is equally distributed throughout the body and is present in sufficient amounts to energize all the cells and tissues of the body.

The chi energy runs through the body in channels called meridians. When working in a healthy manner, these channels distribute the energy evenly throughout the body, sometimes on the surface of the skin and at times deep inside the body in the organs. Disease occurs when the energy flow in a meridian is blocked or stopped. As a result, the internal organs that correspond to the meridians can show symptoms of disease. The meridian flow can be corrected by stimulating the points on the skin surface by hand massage. When the normal flow of energy through the body is resumed, the body is believed to heal itself spontaneously.

Follow the simple instructions and stimulate the acupressure points using finger pressure. It is safe and painless, and does not require the use of needles.

How to Perform Acupressure

Do the acupressure by yourself or with a friend when you are relaxed. Have your room warm and quiet. Make sure your hands are clean and nails trimmed (to avoid bruising yourself). If you tend to have cold hands, put them under warm water.

Work on the side of the body that has the most discomfort. If both sides are equally uncomfortable, choose whichever one you want. Working on one side seems to relieve the symptoms on both sides. Energy or information seems to transfer from one side to the other.

To find the correct acupressure point, look in the photograph accompanying the instructions. Each point corresponds to a specific point on the acupressure meridians. You may massage the points once a day or more during the time that you have symptoms.

Hold each indicated point with a steady pressure for one to three minutes. Apply pressure slowly with the tips or balls of the fingers. Make sure your hand is comfortable. Place several fingers over the area of the point. If you feel resistance or tension in the area to which you are applying pressure, you may want to push a little harder. However, if your hand starts to feel tense or tired, lighten the pressure a bit. The acupressure point may feel somewhat tender. This means the energy pathway or meridian is blocked.

During the treatment, the tenderness in the point should slowly go away. You may also have a subjective feeling of energy radiating from this point into the body. Many patients describe this sensation as very pleasant. Don't worry if you don't feel it—not everyone does. The main goal is relief from your symptoms.

Breathe gently while doing each exercise. As you become more relaxed, your body will respond to the changes in the energy flow.

Exercise 1: Use for Relief of Anxiety and Stress

This exercise helps relieve anxiety, nervous tension, and insomnia. It can also help relieve anxiety coexisting with mitral valve prolapse. It stimulates the entire endocrine system because it involves a powerful point for the pituitary gland. The points in this exercise also help relieve headaches, stiff neck, and stress-related breathing difficulties. This is also an effective exercise for relieving menopause-related hot flashes and hypoglycemia symptoms.

- Sit upright on a chair. Hold each step for 1 to 3 minutes.

- Left hand holds spot located in the slight depression on the top of the head. Right hand holds point directly between the eyebrows where the bridge of the nose meets the forehead.

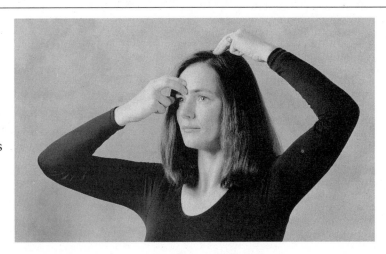

- Right hand holds point in the center of your breastbone, at the level of the heart. Your fingers will fit into the indentations in this bone.

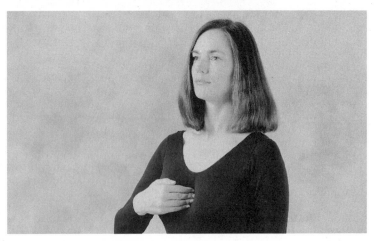

Exercise 2: Use for Relief of Muscle Tension, Stress, and Hypoglycemia

Women who feel anxious and stressed often suffer from tight muscles. This important sequence of points helps relieve upper body tension. The neck and shoulders generally carry a great deal of tension. Tightness in this area can act as a bottleneck and impede the energy flow of the entire body. Thus, this sequence energizes the entire body, relieving fatigue and burnout as well as relieving anxiety and nervous tension. The points in this sequence strengthen the immune system and also include a major treatment point for hypoglycemia.

- Hold each step 1 to 3 minutes. You will begin in a lying-down position and then sit upright on a chair.

- Fold a towel in half lengthwise. Lie down on your back and place the towel underneath your upper back between your shoulder blades, applying pressure to an important pressure point. Relax in this position for 1 to 3 minutes.

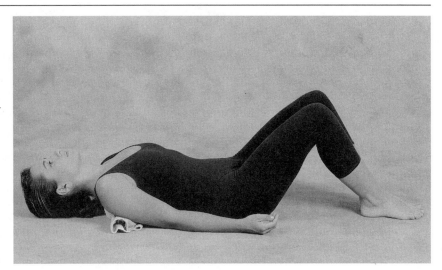

- Now sit up. Left hand holds a point at the top of the shoulder blade, 1 to 2 inches to the side of the spine. The point is between the shoulder blade and the spine. It may feel firm and resistant.

  Right hand holds the same point on the right side.

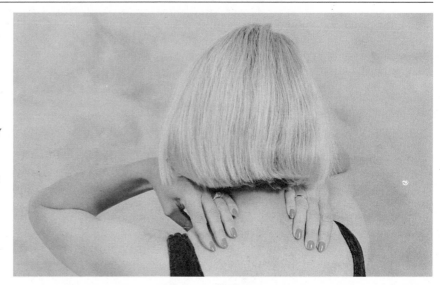

- Left hand holds a point slightly to the back of the top of the shoulder where the neck meets the shoulder.

  Right hand holds the same point on the right side.

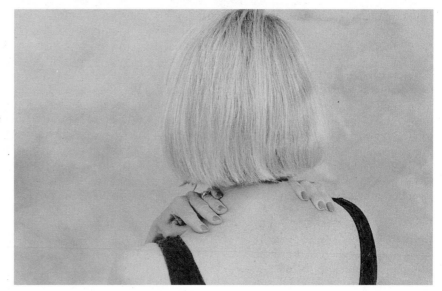

- Left hand holds the point
  halfway on the neck;
  fingers rest on the muscle
  next to the spine.

  Right hand holds the same
  point on the right side.

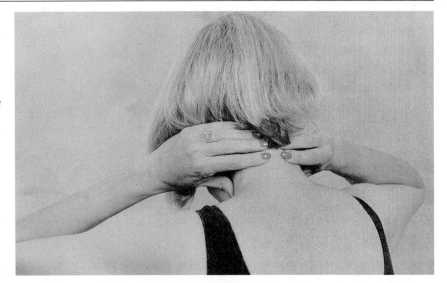

- Left hand holds the point
  underneath the base of the
  skull, 1 to 2 inches out
  from the spine. Your
  fingers will feel a hollow
  spot at this point.

  Right hand holds the point
  on the right side.

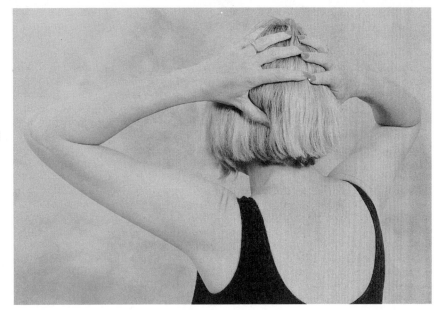

Exercise 3: Use for Relief of Insomnia

This exercise helps relieve insomnia and anxiety. In Oriental medicine, these points are called "joyful sleep" and "calm sleep."

- Sit comfortably and hold these points for 1 to 3 minutes.

- Left hand holds the point on the inside of the right ankle. This point is located in the indentation directly below the inner ankle bone.

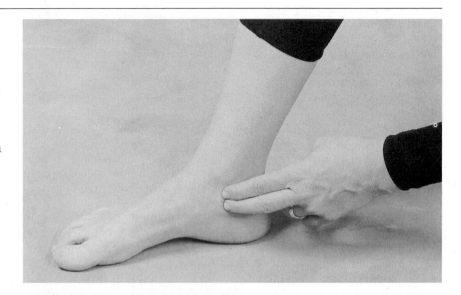

- Right hand holds the point located in the indentation below the right outer ankle.

  Repeat this exercise holding the points on the left foot.

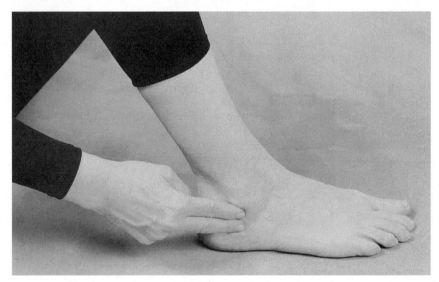

Exercise 4: Use to Relieve Chest Tension

This exercise relieves chest tension and shallow breathing caused by anxiety. It also involves a point that reduces hypoglycemia symptoms.

- Sit comfortably. Hold each point 1 to 3 minutes.

- Left hand holds the point on the outer part of the chest. This point is located three fingerwidths below the collarbone.

  Right hand holds the same point on the right side.

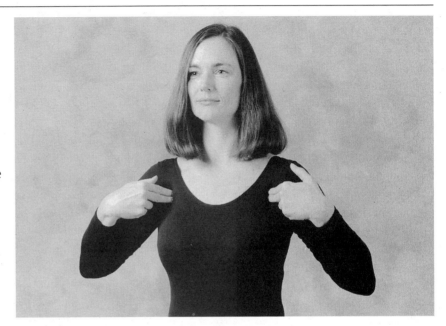

- Left hand holds a point on the right hand below the base of the thumb, in the wrist groove.

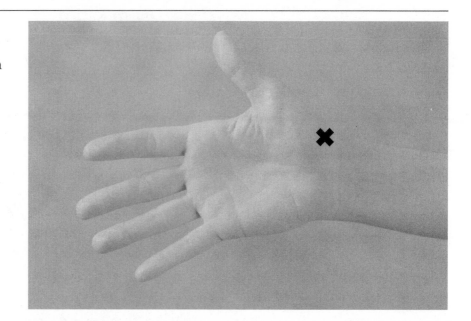

- Left hand holds a point on the palm side of the right hand in the center of the pad below the thumb.

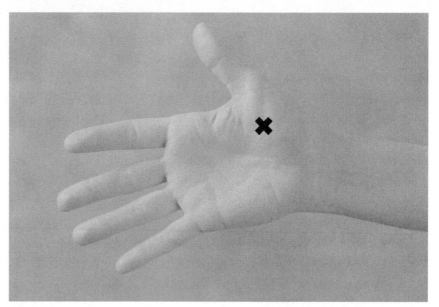

Exercise 5: Use for Relief of Digestive Tension

This powerful energy point is one of the most important in Oriental medicine. It helps relieve digestive problems due to nervous tension and anxiety. It is also used to quickly diminish fatigue and improve energy and endurance. It has traditionally been used by athletes to tone and strengthen the muscles as well as increase stamina.

- Sit upright on a chair. Hold the point for 1 to 3 minutes.

- Left hand holds a point below right knee. Locate this point with right hand, measuring four finger-widths below the kneecap toward the outside of the shinbone. It is sensitive to the touch in many people.

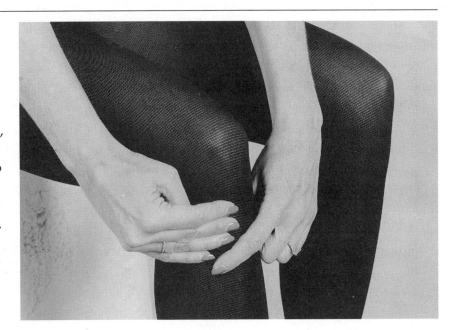

Exercise 6: Relieves PMS and Menstrual-Related Anxiety

This exercise relieves PMS symptoms and menstrual cramps by balancing points on the bladder meridian. This meridian relieves symptoms by balancing the energy of the female reproductive tract. Oriental medicine uses these points to relieve anxiety, fear, and exhaustion related to PMS, cramps, and other reproductive problems.

- Sit on the floor and prop your back against a wall or a heavy piece of furniture. Hold each step for 1 to 3 minutes.

- Alternative Method: Lie on the floor and put your lower legs over the seat of a chair. Follow the exercise from that position.

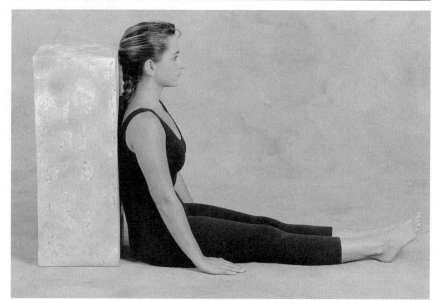

- Place right hand 1 inch above the waist on the muscle to the left side of the spine (muscle will feel firm and ropelike). Place left hand behind crease of the right knee.

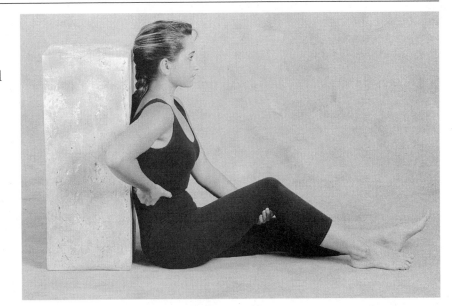

- Right hand stays in the same position. Left hand is placed on the center of the back of the right calf. This is just below the fullest part of the calf.

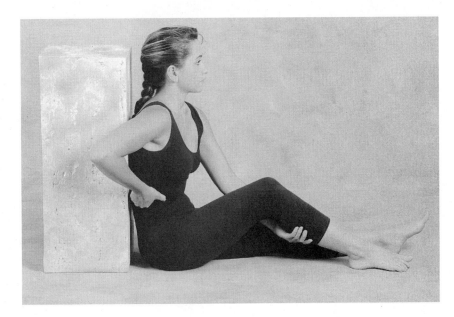

- Right hand remains 1 inch above the waist on the muscle to the side of the spine. Left hand is placed just below the ankle bone on the outside of the right heel.

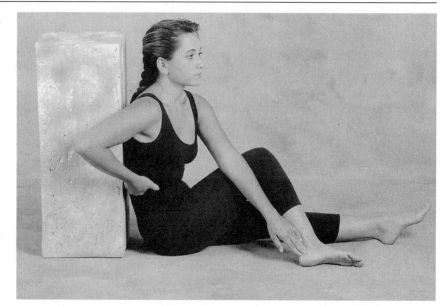

- Right hand stays in the same position. Left hand holds the front and back of the right little toe at the nail.

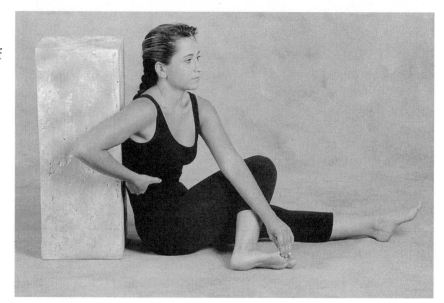

Exercise 7: Relieves Menstrual Stress and Fatigue

This exercise helps relieve menstrual anxiety and depression, helpful to women suffering from significant stress in their lives. It helps relieve hot flashes related to the onset of menopause, as well as breathing difficulties caused by anxiety. The sequence of points relieves fatigue that many women experience for up to several days prior to the onset of their menstrual period. The second step in this sequence has traditionally been forbidden for use by pregnant women after their first trimester.

- Sit up and prop your back against a chair. Hold each step for 1 to 3 minutes.

- Right hand holds a point at the base of the ball of the right foot. This point is located between the two pads of the foot.

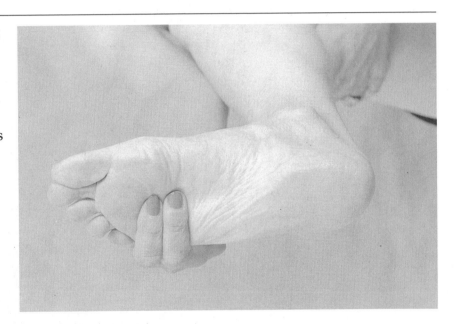

- Left hand holds the point midway between the inside of the right ankle bone and the Achilles tendon. The Achilles tendon is located at the back of the ankle.

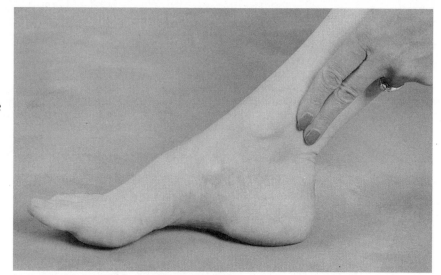

- Left hand holds a point below right knee, located four fingerwidths below the kneecap toward the outside of the shinbone. It is sensitive to the touch in many people.

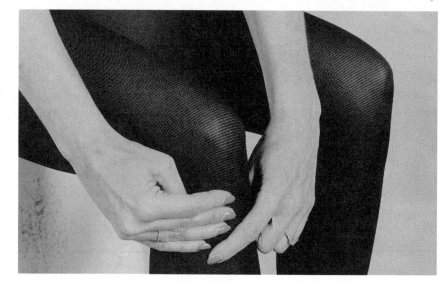

Exercise 8: Use to Balance the Thyroid Gland

These points help balance the thyroid gland and normalize thyroid function. They also promote healthy skin tone and color.

- Sit or lie in a comfortable position. Hold each step for 1 to 3 minutes.

- Left hand holds a point in the indentation behind the ear lobe.

- Left hand holds a point directly below the ear lobe and behind the jawbone.

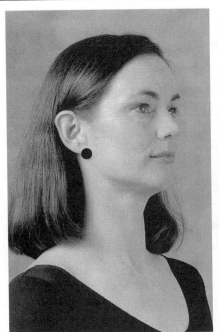 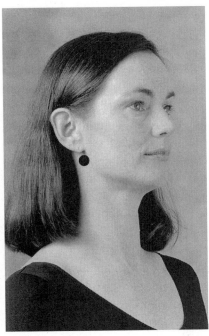

Exercise 9: Use to Balance the Thyroid Gland

This exercise balances the thyroid gland. A hyperactive gland can cause anxiety and nervousness.

- Sit upright on a chair. Hold each step for 1 to 3 minutes.

- Hands wrap around shoulders with thumbs pressing gently into both sides on top of collarbone.

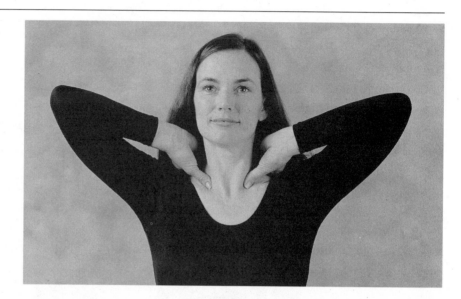

- Fingers are in back. Press against upper shoulders and shoulder blade area.

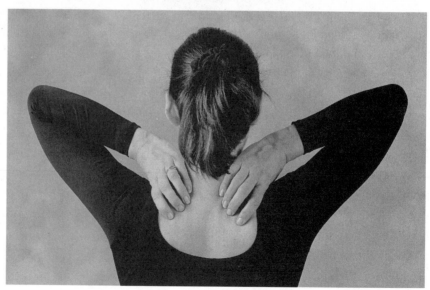

Exercise 10: Use for Relief of Food Addiction

This exercise helps relieve food cravings and addictions for foods that worsen anxiety and nervous tension. This includes chocolate, sugar, and caffeine. This exercise also helps relieve anxiety and emotional stress, which often worsen digestive problems. Use this point on an empty stomach prior to eating. Do not hold this point deeply.

- Sit or lie in a comfortable position. Hold this point for 1 to 3 minutes.

- Right hand holds a point in the midline of the body, halfway between the bottom of the breast bone and the navel.

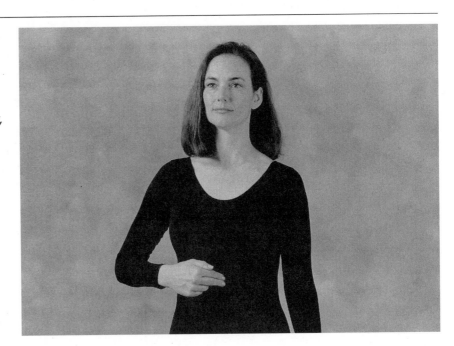

11

Treating Anxiety with Drugs

Though this book has emphasized the importance and effectiveness of self help techniques for the treatment of anxiety and stress, medication also has a proper place in some circumstances. This is particularly true when symptoms of anxiety are severe. Medication may then be necessary in order to attain adequate symptom relief for the patient in distress. This will be equally true for you whether you suffer from emotionally based causes of anxiety or have certain physical problems that cause anxiety, such as PMS, menopause, hyperthyroidism, and mitral valve prolapse.

Drugs as Appropriate Therapy

During my 20 years of medical practice, I have tended to use drugs as a second line of treatment. I approach the use of drugs cautiously because of their powerful chemical effects on the body and potential for causing toxic side effects. My preference is to use the safer and gentler natural therapies such as diet, supplemental nutrients, stress-reduction techniques, deep breathing exercises, counseling, and physical exercises as my first line of treatment whenever possible.

When Drugs Are Appropriate

Sometimes, however, the use of drugs may be an absolute necessity for the well-being of the patient. This is often the case when the symptoms are so severe that they do not respond completely to the natural therapies. Examples are anxiety, phobias, and panic attacks of such frequency and severity that they will not allow a woman to function and carry out her necessary daily activities, whether performing a job or taking care of children. Also, if the anxiety condition is causing too much emotional pain and distress, then medication is indicated, at least on a short-term basis.

Similarly, a woman with severe menopause-related anxiety, mood swings, and associated symptoms, such as hot flashes or night sweats caused by hormonal deficiency, may require hormonal replacement therapy. This may be necessary to give her the relief she needs and get her back to a level of emotional and physiological comfort.

Often, to obtain the best results in treating anxiety and stress of all types, I combine the medication with natural therapies. This gives a woman the full range of available treatment options. It also emphasizes prevention as well as immediate symptom relief.

Using Drugs Safely and Effectively

When using drugs for the treatment of anxiety, I always try to prescribe medication only for short-term use and at the lowest therapeutic dose. Unfortunately, drug addiction and unpleasant side effects are real possibilities with the long-term use of many anxiety-reducing drugs, particularly at high doses. The judicious and careful use of these medications reduces the risk of unpleasant side effects, as well as the withdrawal symptoms that can occur when drugs are discontinued.

Before embarking on a medication program, make sure you understand both the risks and benefits of the medications that you are considering. Discuss with your physician the potential side effects and any contraindications to normal activities when using these drugs. For example, if a drug causes sedative effects, you should not attempt to drive a car when these side effects are pronounced. Find out how long your physician plans to keep you on medication and after what time period it will be discontinued to avoid withdrawal effects. Your physician should have a good plan in mind when beginning a program that includes medication.

Before you start on medication, provide all information to your physician that could affect the use of a particular drug. Pertinent information includes data about *any* allergies or unusual reactions that you might have to drugs or any other substances, such as foods, preservatives, or dyes. For example, if you have mitral valve prolapse, you will need to use antibiotics prophylactically before dental work or surgery. Be sure to notify your physician if you are currently taking any other prescription or over-the-counter medications. This will help prevent potentially dangerous drug interaction effects. Inform your doctor if you are pregnant or breast-feeding, because the use of medications can be dangerous to the fetus or nursing infant. If you develop any new medical problem while you are using any of the following prescription drugs, inform your physician immediately.

If you find communication with your physician difficult or feel uncomfortable talking about your concerns, I suggest that you find another physician with whom you do feel comfortable. The decision about whether to use a particular medication requires a mutual decision on the part of the patient and physician, exchanging full information about the patient's condition and the risks and benefits of the drug. Such matters can be best discussed in a positive patient-doctor relationship.

In the following section of this chapter, I describe the drugs used most commonly for both the emotional and physical causes of anxiety and stress. This should provide you with useful information when making a decision with your physician about drug therapy.

Prescription Drugs

Four major types of prescription drugs can be useful in relieving anxiety, stress, and panic symptoms; benzodiazepine tranquilizers and sedatives, antidepressants, beta-blockers, and an antianxiety drug (buspirone hydrochloride). I discuss their uses as well as their side effects.

Benzodiazepine Tranquilizers and Sedatives

Benzodiazepines are among the most commonly used medications for treating anxiety. They decrease anxiety by depressing the central nervous system. All have sedative properties, too, depending on the dosage. Pharmaceutical companies have developed and isolated more than two thousand benzodiazepine formulas and tested over one hundred of them for antianxiety properties. Benzodiazepines are divided into two groups: tranquilizers and sedatives.

Of the first group, benzodiazepine tranquilizers, Xanax™ (alprazolam), Librium™ (chlordiazepoxide hydrochloride), Valium™ (diazepam), Tranxene™ (clorazepate), and Klonopin™ (clonazepam) are most commonly prescribed for acute anxiety on a short-term basis and, in lower doses, for panic disorders on a longer-term basis. Physicians and psychiatrists also prescribe these drugs to treat women with PMS- and menopause-related anxiety as well as women with eating disorders, especially food addiction coexisting with anxiety.

In high doses, the tranquilizers behave like sedatives; thus, they can also be used to induce sleep. Certain tranquilizers like Valium™ reduce muscle tension and spasm, which is sometimes aggravated in women who suffer from excessive anxiety and stress. Other tranquilizers like Librium™ may be combined with a second antispasmodic drug to create drugs like Librax™, which reduces both anxiety and smooth muscle spasm. Conditions like irritable bowel syndrome, commonly triggered by anxiety and stress, respond well to these combinations. Certain of the tranquilizers are also used to treat the anxiety associated with alcohol withdrawal; these include Serax™ (oxazepam), Tranxene™, Librium™, and Valium™. The last two drugs can be given intravenously to alcoholics, a benefit for people who react to the oral drugs with nausea and vomiting.

The second group, benzodiazepine sedatives ("sleeping pills"), includes Dalmane™ (flurazepam), Halcion™ (triazolam), Restoril™ (temazepam), and Ativan™ (lorazepam). These sedatives are very effective in inducing a state of deep and refreshing sleep when first started. They are useful on a short-term basis and for women with severe acute anxiety as well as insomnia caused by menopause and PMS episodes. With continuing use, however, the patient develops a tolerance to the drugs and the doses need to be gradually increased. This brings with it the risk of increased side effects as well as withdrawal symptoms when therapy is discontinued. Thus, these drugs should preferably be used only for short courses of therapy.

Because all the benzodiazepines have similar mechanisms of action, they differ mainly in how long they stay in your body (called their "half-life") after the liver breaks down the components into chemical metabolites. The metabolites are the form in which they're excreted from your body. Some benzodiazepines like Valium™ and Dalmane™ have long half-lives, while Xanax™ and Halcion™ tend to have short half-lives and are excreted rapidly.

Benzodiazepine tranquilizers and sedatives have similar side effects including drowsiness, lethargy, fatigue, and "morning hangover." Occasionally, paradoxic reactions can occur within the first few weeks of therapy. These reactions are characterized by an increase in anxiety, irritability, rage, insomnia, and even hallucinations.

When benzodiazepine tranquilizers and sedatives are prescribed for long periods of time (more than several months), withdrawal symptoms may occur on discontinuing therapy. This is because the long-term use of these drugs can result in physical and psychological addiction. Tolerance can develop and the dosages have to be increased over time to continue to get a therapeutic effect. Abrupt withdrawal can produce symptoms similar to alcohol withdrawal. Milder withdrawal symptoms include insomnia, weakness, and anxiety. More severe symptoms include seizures and delirium. Ideally, withdrawal of benzodiazepines should take place gradually over a two- to four-week period.

In summary, the benzodiazepine medications have a wide range of uses for the treatment of anxiety, irritability, insomnia, and muscle tension caused by both emotional and physical problems, including acute anxiety, panic disorders, PMS, menopause, food addiction, and alcohol abuse. However, because of side effects and drug tolerances that increase with elevations in the dose, and because of the problem of drug dependency that can develop over time, these drugs should be prescribed only for short periods of time. Also, they are not curative. Eighty percent of women report recurrence of their anxiety symptoms once the drugs are stopped. Thus, while these medications can relieve symptoms temporarily, a combination of natural self help therapies and counseling is needed to prevent a recurrence of anxiety symptoms on a long-term basis.

Antidepressants

Antidepressants are the medications most commonly used to treat depression if it coexists with anxiety. They are also used to treat panic attacks or agoraphobia with panic attacks. Antidepressants are also commonly prescribed for women with PMS and menopause who suffer from mood symptoms.

The antidepressants used today are primarily tricyclic antidepressants, commonly known as "mood elevators." These produce both an antidepressant and mild tranquilizing effect. Because it takes some time to build up to a therapeutic effect once treatment is initiated, there is a dangerous period of time before the drug takes hold when the patient may remain depressed and become suicidal. However, after two to three weeks of treatment, 80 percent of depressed and anxious patients notice an elevation of mood, increased alertness, and improvement in appetite. Common tricyclic medications include Elavil™ (amitriptyline), Tofranil™ (imipramine), Sinequan™ (doxepin), Aventyl™ (nortriptyline), and Norpramin™ (desipramine). While the actual mechanism of action is not known, it is thought that depression is relieved by elevating the levels of neurotransmitters like serotonin and norepinephrine. These are chemicals present in the brain that regulate mood, personality, sleep, and appetite. Many women with depression may lack adequate levels of these neurotransmitters.

Which antidepressants are best suited for panic episodes, agoraphobia, and anxiety coexisting with depression varies from person to person. The efficiency of any antidepressant depends on each individual's body chemistry. As a result, the patient may have to try several antidepressants to find the one that produces the best therapeutic effect.

Side effects of these drugs are fairly common. In fact, as many as one-quarter of all patients stop therapy with these drugs because of the unpleasant side effects. Many women using antidepressants will initially complain of dry mouth, blurred vision, constipation, drowsiness, or even anxiety and agitation. These symptoms tend to fade in intensity after the first few weeks of taking the medication; sometimes they are minimized by initiating therapy at very low doses. Other side effects include the development of shakiness or tremors in the hands; these occur in 10 percent of patients. Numbness and tingling in the arms and legs are also reported occasionally.

Unlike the benzodiazepines, antidepressants are not physically addictive, so the threat of developing withdrawal symptoms is not an issue. However, some women become psychologically addicted to the antidepressants and may have a difficult time weaning themselves off medication.

Once the antidepressants are stopped, the symptoms may recur, but less frequently than is experienced by women taking benzodiazepines. Recurrence rate runs between 25 and 50 percent (contrasted with approximately 80 to 90 percent for benzodiazepines). Thus, use of these medications for at least six months may also help prevent the recurrence of depression for a long period of time.

Several other antidepressants unrelated to the tricyclic class are also currently on the market. These include medications such as Prozac™ (fluoxetine hydrochloride) and Desyrel™ (trazodone hydrochloride). Like the tricyclic medications, both of these drugs appear to exert their effects on the nervous system by blocking the mechanism involved in the uptake of neurotransmitters, thereby elevating the levels of serotonin. Even though the literature suggests these drugs cause fewer side effects, they must be used cautiously. The side effects are like those of the tricyclic antidepressants and include headaches, drowsiness, fatigue, nervousness, insomnia, change in sex drive, nausea, diarrhea, sweating, rashes, and muscle aches.

In summary, antidepressants can produce much benefit in the short- to intermediate-term treatment of anxiety coexisting with depression, panic episodes, and agoraphobia. They're also useful for the treatment of PMS- and menopause-related depression. While side effects are common and psychological dependency can develop, physical dependency is not a problem. Also, in some women the recurrence of depression is prevented or at least delayed once treatment is stopped.

Beta Blockers

These drugs are primarily used to treat conditions triggered by hyperactivity of the sympathetic nervous system. This is the part of the nervous system that triggers the fight-or-flight response, with increased heart and pulse rate. Beta blockers such as Inderal™ (propranolol hydrochloride) help reduce nervous system hyperactivity by blocking the transmission of nerve impulses to the beta-type receptors of the sympathetic nervous system. These receptors are found in abundance in the nerves that control the heart muscle. By slowing down the heart rate, these drugs relieve such stress-sensitive problems as cardiac arrhythmia (irregular or overly fast heartbeat), high blood pressure, and migraine headaches. Inderal is also commonly used to treat anxiety, particularly when accompanied by physical symptoms such as rapid heartbeat or heart palpitations. It is particularly useful when taken as a single dose to relieve anxiety symptoms that may precede a stressful situation like public speaking, examinations, or a job interview. Women with mitral valve prolapse are more prone to panic attacks than the general population, for reasons that are not yet understood. In women with this condition, the use of Inderal™ can help to control rapid or irregular heartbeat and anxiety episodes.

The use of Inderal™ should be avoided altogether or monitored carefully in women with pre-existing congestive heart failure or asthma, because the use of this drug may worsen these conditions. Inderal™ may help relieve the symptoms of hyperthyroidism, a physical cause of anxiety. However, it should be used carefully because it may mask clinical signs of conditions such as tachycardia, making it difficult to evaluate the severity of underlying conditions. While slowing the heart rate is beneficial for women with hyperthyroidism, discontinuing the Inderal™ may worsen the symptoms and put the patient at risk of precipitating a thyroid crisis.

Women with anxiety symptoms who do not have these potentially dangerous preexisting conditions may use Inderal™ with reasonable safety. Common side effects include excessive slowing of the heart rate, lowering of blood pressure, light-headedness, fatigue, weakness, drowsiness, nausea, vomiting, and abdominal cramping. If Inderal is prescribed on a regular basis, withdrawal symptoms can occur, so drug use should be stopped gradually over a sufficient period of time.

Antianxiety

BuSpar™ (buspirone hydrochloride) is a relatively new antianxiety drug that has two definite benefits over benzodiazepines and other sedatives. First, it does not cause excessive levels of sedation, so the potentially debilitating side effect of drowsiness is decreased. Second, it is not addictive, so women using BuSpar™ do not run the risk of becoming dependent on this drug or having to go through a potentially uncomfortable withdrawal period in order to discontinue it. As a result, some physicians now favor it over traditional drugs such as Xanax™ for regular use in treating generalized anxiety. It is also useful for treating the anxiety component when anxiety and depression coexist. It is less useful, however, in treating panic attacks and is usually not used for anxiety or tension created by the stress of everyday living.

Though BuSpar™ is a relatively safe drug, it should not be used with antidepressant medication belonging to the monoamine oxidase inhibitor (MAO inhibitor) classification. Interaction of these two drugs may cause an elevation in blood pressure. Also, even though BuSpar™ has been found to be less sedating than other antianxiety drugs, a woman taking it should avoid operating an automobile until she is sure that the drug does not affect her mental and motor performance. Nervous system side effects such as drowsiness, dizziness, nervousness, and insomnia of sufficient severity to necessitate discontinuing use of the drug were seen in 3.4 percent of 2200 women studied in a clinical trial. This trial was done during the preapproval stage of testing to gather the necessary data so that the drug could be sold in the United States. In the same clinical trial, 1.2 percent of the women tested experienced digestive disturbances such as nausea severe enough to necessitate discontinuing the drug. Other reported side effects include chest pain, dream disturbances, tinnitus (ringing in the ears), sore throat, and nasal congestion. The side effects occur in a relatively small number of patients using the drug, however. For women who tolerate the drug well, the lack of physical dependence or potential for drug abuse make it a drug of choice for the treatment of generalized anxiety.

Drugs for PMS

Several drug therapies are available for the treatment of PMS-related anxiety, mood swings, and increased sensitivity to stress. These include progesterone as well as mood-altering drugs like the benzodiazepine tranquilizers and antidepressants. I discuss the use of progesterone here. For information on tranquilizers and antidepressants, see the preceding discussion.

Progesterone

Progesterone is a hormone secreted by the ovaries after ovulation, present along with estrogen during the second half of the menstrual cycle. Since PMS also begins after ovulation, many suspect that imbalances in the levels of estrogen and progesterone cause PMS, particularly the emotional symptoms. (More than 80 percent of women with PMS complain of anxiety and mood swings from several days to two weeks each month.) Since both estrogen and progesterone affect brain chemistry as well as mood, this is a particularly interesting hypothesis. Excessive levels of estrogen are linked to anxiety and irritability, while progesterone has a sedative effect on the brain. Progesterone also increases the brain's output of its own opiates, such as beta endorphins, which help promote a sense of emotional well-being. When the balance between the two female hormones is tipped in favor of one hormone or the other, emotional symptoms can occur. This certainly occurs in younger women on the birth control pill or in menopausal women on hormonal replacement therapy. Symptoms of anxiety and edginess or depression and fatigue can occur if the hormonal mix provided by the pill is poorly matched to the patient's body type. Different dosages or formulas may have to be tried until the mix is right for a particular patient.

Unfortunately, the research studies done on this issue show contradictory data. Is PMS actually caused by a progesterone deficiency or imbalance, or does progesterone even help relieve this condition in controlled clinical studies? The negative medical research findings contradict the experiences of many women with PMS who have used progesterone therapy. Many women feel progesterone is the only medical treatment that finally helped to eradicate their anxiety. Often their physicians have prescribed a whole range of mood-altering drugs in order to relieve the more severe anxiety and mood swing symptoms without positive results. When they then try progesterone, many women obtain symptom relief. In fact, progesterone is currently the most widely prescribed therapy for the treatment of PMS. A recent study showed that 70 percent of the physicians in the United States who treat PMS use progesterone therapy.

In my practice, I prefer to use progesterone as a second line of treatment to accompany the natural therapies like diet, nutritional supplements, and stress management, and only if the severity of the symptoms warrants drug use. My own impression has been that progesterone does help to reduce PMS symptoms in some women.

Start progesterone therapy three days before the onset of PMS symptoms. For example, if PMS symptoms normally begin five days before your menstrual period, you should start taking progesterone eight days before the expected onset of your period. Progesterone is most commonly available as a rectal or vaginal suppository or as a tablet to be taken orally. However, nasal drops and even progesterone skin creams are occasionally used. Suppositories are commonly prescribed in 200-mg dosages, with most women using a total of 400 to 800 mg of progesterone per day during their treatment period. However, lower doses or doses as high as 1200 mg a day may give the best therapeutic results for some patients.

Side effects of progesterone therapy are quite rare; they include local irritation of the rectal or vulvar mucosa caused by the medium in which the progesterone is mixed, leakage of the progesterone from the vagina, and a slight increase in the incidence of yeast vaginitis. In women with irregular menstrual cycles, high doses of progesterone may delay the onset of menstruation.

This can be remedied by simply stopping the progesterone; menstrual bleeding will follow soon after.

Drugs for Menopause

Estrogen and progestin (a synthetic form of progesterone) therapy is usually the drug treatment of choice for menopause-related anxiety and edginess. However, the use of tranquilizers and antidepressants may occasionally be necessary to help a woman through the more unstable phases of menopause. This is particularly true during the early stages of menopause when the hormonal swings can be erratic and abrupt. Menopausal women under stress are particularly susceptible to wide mood swings as their hormonal levels drop from the higher levels of the active reproductive years to the lower levels typical of the postmenopausal period. These women may need both hormones and mood stabilizing drugs. I discuss the use of estrogen and progestin therapy here; for more information on the benefits and side effects of benzodiazepine tranquilizers and sedatives as well as antidepressants, please refer to the earlier section of this chapter, "Prescription Drugs."

Hormonal Replacement Therapy

The issue of whether to use hormones or not is a question that most menopausal women pursue with their own physician as well as with friends and through reading materials. The use of estrogen is very much in the news as so many baby-boomers are beginning the transition into menopause. Statistically, estrogen and progestin use is much lower than most women suspect. Only 15 percent of women in the menopause and postmenopause age group actually use hormonal replacement therapy (HRT). The women who choose not to use HRT often do so because their symptoms are mild or absent or they have many concerns about the possible immediate and long-term side effects that could occur with the use of hormones. For women with moderate to severe anxiety, irritability, depression, fatigue, and insomnia related to menopausal hormonal changes, the use of HRT can be very beneficial.

Many menopausal women find that hormonal replacement therapy helps their moods and gives their energy level a tremendous boost. Many of my patients have reported not only relief from hot flashes and vaginal dryness, but also reduction in anxiety and improved sex drive. Depression, the blues, and fatigue are often eradicated, as are insomnia and irritability.

You can take estrogen in pill form, as a vaginal cream, as a skin patch, or by injection. There are many brands on the market, generally composed of combinations of two types of estrogen that occur naturally in your body: estrone and estradiol. Estrone is the main type of estrogen that your body makes after menopause, while estradiol is present in greater amounts during your menstrual years.

Both synthetic and naturally derived estrogen are available. The most popular brand is Premarin™ (conjugated estrogen tablets), which comes from the urine of pregnant mares and contains a natural mixture of estrogen, including estrone. Other popular brands include Ogen™ (estropipate tablets), which contains estrone, and Estrace™ (estradiol tablets), which contains estradiol.

If you take estrogen as a pill, it is usually administered daily from the first to the twenty-fifth day of the month. About a week after taking the last pill, bleeding similar to a menstrual period will occur unless, of course, a woman has had a hysterectomy. A progestin such as Provera™ is usually added for 10 to 14 days at the end of each 25-day course of estrogen because research studies indicate that it protects women from developing uterine cancer. For that reason, most doctors today prescribe a combination of estrogen and progestin for menopause symptoms. Common brands of progestins on the market include Provera™ (medroxyprogesterone acetate), Amen™ (medroxyprogesterone acetate), and Norlutin™ (norethindrone tablets).

Because of the possible side effects of using hormones, most physicians prescribe the lowest dose of both estrogen and progestins that relieves symptoms. Much higher doses were used several decades ago, both in estrogen replacement therapy and in birth control pills, but the current trend is definitely toward smaller doses of hormones to achieve the same beneficial effects. Women with a history of uterine or breast cancer, active fibroid tumors, endometriosis, liver or gall bladder disease, and vascular problems should avoid hormonal replacement therapy. Unfortunately, progestins like Provera™ can worsen fatigue and depression in susceptible women. Women with coexisting anxiety and depression should use them cautiously.

Drugs for Hyperthyroidism

Excessive secretion of thyroid hormone may cause symptoms of anxiety and nervousness. While these symptoms are usually accompanied by physical symptoms such as sweating, weight loss, loose bowel movements, and rapid heartbeat, initially distinguishing between emotional causes of anxiety and hyperthyroidism in a particular patient may be difficult. Once the diagnosis has been determined by thyroid function testing, the focus of treatment will be on halting the thyroid's excessive secretion of hormone. Suppressing the thyroid either surgically or through drugs is the treatment. Drug therapy for the suppression of the thyroid gland is discussed here.

Propylthiouracil

Propylthiouracil is an antithyroid drug that blocks the production of thyroid hormone within the gland itself. Propylthiouracil does not destroy hormone that has already been produced. As a result, it can take up to four to six weeks for elevated levels of thyroid hormone to return to normal. Once the thyroid level is within the normal range, the patient can be placed on a lower maintenance dose of the drug to keep the thyroid levels from rising again. However, thyroid function tests must be monitored periodically to make sure that the levels don't fall too low, producing hypothyroidism. Alternatively, some physicians prefer to use propylthiouracil at higher doses until the patient's thyroid hormone drops to levels below the normal range. At this point, thyroid replacement therapy is instituted to bring the patient's thyroid levels back to normal.

Propylthiouracil is the treatment of choice in young women and children because it allows reproductive options to remain intact. It provides an alternative to surgical removal of the thyroid gland and avoids the risks and potential postoperative complications of surgery. Other than hypothyroidism, which can be minimized with careful monitoring, side effects include a skin rash, which develops in 5 percent of patients. Other, less frequent side effects include headaches, muscle and joint aches, enlargements of lymph glands in the neck, and loss of the sense of taste.

The long-term use of the drug seems to help prevent recurrence of hyperthyroidism. In patients treated between 18 and 24 months with propylthiouracil, between 50 and 70 percent have no recurrence of the disease after the drug dosage is slowly decreased and finally discontinued. Women having a recurrence after drug cessation may have further treatment with propylthiouracil, radioactive iodine, or surgery.

Radioactive Iodine

In some cases, a radioactive isotope of iodine is administered simply by having the patient drink water treated with radioactive iodine. Colorless and tasteless, the water treated with radiation is quite dangerous to the thyroid gland. The radioactive iodine is selectively absorbed into the thyroid gland in high concentrations. It then acts to destroy the thyroid gland while posing no damage to other tissues in the body. As a result, excessive thyroid hormone levels fall. The hormones often slowly fall to the hypothyroid level within a few years of treatment. Since the hormone-producing cells of the thyroid are essentially destroyed, thyroid replacement therapy becomes necessary.

Therapy with radioactive iodine is generally used in women over 30 who have no further wish to bear children. This is because the radiation may be a possible cause of genetic damage. There is also an increased risk of the development of cancer with the use of this drug. Like propylthiouracil, it does offer a nonsurgical approach to the treatment of hyperthyroidism. Even with its potential side effects and permanent destruction of the thyroid gland itself, this alternative to surgery can prevent much debilitating wear and tear on the patient.

In summary, a wide variety of drugs offer the possibility of real symptom relief for emotional and physical causes of severe anxiety. All drugs run the risk of causing both short-term and long-term side effects, however. Before beginning any drug therapy, a woman should discuss possible risks and benefits with her physician. This allows for the best possible choice of medication, and the smallest chance of adverse side effects.

Prescription Drugs

Anxiety and depression
- Benzodiazepine tranquilizers
- Benzodiazepine sedatives
- Antidepressants
- Beta-blockers
- Antianxiety

Food addiction
- Antidepressants

PMS
- Progesterone
- Benzodiazepine tranquilizers
- Antidepressants

Menopause
- Estrogen and progesterone (either natural or synthetic)
- Benzodiazepine tranquilizers
- Benzodiazepine sedatives
- Antidepressants

Hyperthyroidism
- Propylthiouracil
- Radioactive iodine
- Thyroid replacement therapy
- Beta-blockers

Mitral valve prolapse
- Beta-blockers

12

How to Put Your Program Together

Anxiety and Stress has given you a complete self help program to prevent and relieve your symptoms. I have included many treatment options to work with as you put your personal program together. Try the therapies that feel most comfortable. You may find that certain exercises or stress-reduction routines feel better than others. If so, practice the ones that bring the greatest sense of relief for your particular symptoms.

Don't get bogged down in details. Always keep in mind that your ultimate goal is relief of your anxiety symptoms and a general improvement in your overall health and well-being. I usually recommend beginning any self help program slowly so you can comfortably become accustomed to the lifestyle changes. People differ in their ability to adjust to major lifestyle changes. Though some of my patients like to eliminate their old, unhealthy habits as quickly as possible, many other women find such rapid changes in their long-term habits to be too stressful. Find the pace that works for you.

Enjoy the program. I always tell my patients to regard their self help program as an enjoyable adventure. The exercise and stress-reduction routines should give you a sense of emotional balance and well-being. The menus and food selections I've recommended in this book provide you with an opportunity to try delicious and healthful new foods.

As you do the program, don't set up unrealistic or overly strict expectations for yourself. You don't have to be perfect to get great results. Just follow the guidelines of the program as well as you can and as your schedule permits.

You will not be courting disaster if you occasionally forget to take your vitamins or don't have time to exercise on a particular day. Don't be discouraged if you can't follow the dietary recommendations on vacations, holidays, and birthdays. Periodically review the guidelines outlined in this book and continue to adapt your lifestyle to the healthful suggestions that I've shared with you. Over time you will notice many beneficial changes.

Be your own feedback system. Your body will tell you if you are on the right track and if what you are doing is making you feel better. It will also tell you if your current diet and emotional stresses are making your symptoms worse. Remember that even moderate changes in your habits can make significant differences.

The Anxiety Workbook

Fill out the workbook section of this book. The questionnaires will help you determine which areas in your life have contributed the most to your symptoms and need the most improvement. Then, by reviewing the workbook every month or two as you follow the self help program, you will see the areas in which you are making the most progress, with both symptom relief and initiation of healthier lifestyle habits. The workbook can provide feedback in an organized and easy-to-use manner.

Diet and Nutritional Supplements

I recommend that you make all nutritional changes gradually. Many women find breakfast the easiest meal to change because it is simple and often eaten at home. To change your other meals and snacks, periodically review the lists of foods to eliminate and those to emphasize. Each month, pick a few foods that you are willing to eliminate from your diet. In their place, try the foods that help prevent and relieve anxiety. The recipes and menus in Chapter 4 should be very helpful; use the meal plans as guidelines while you restructure your diet to suit your needs.

Vitamins, minerals, essential fatty acids, and herbal supplements will help complete your nutritional program and speed up the healing process. Most women find these a very important part of their self help program.

Stress Reduction and Breathing Exercises

The stress-reduction and breathing exercises can play an important role in facilitating your emotional and physical healing process. These exercises have been designed to induce a state of peace, calm, and relaxation, as well as reinforce new ways of handling stress. When practiced on a regular basis, they also help build confidence and self-esteem. The visualization exercises can help you set a blueprint in your mind for optimal health; this enables your body and mind to work together in harmony.

Begin by trying all the stress-reduction and breathing exercises listed in this book. Choose the combination that works best for you. Practice stress management on a regular basis and be aware of your habitual breathing patterns. Both these techniques will help you relax and release tensions.

You do not need to spend enormous amounts of time on these exercises. Allocate 15 to 30 minutes each day, depending on the flexibility of your schedule; even 10 minutes out of your daily schedule can be helpful. You may find that the quietest times for you are early in the morning before you get out of bed, or late at night before going to sleep; or, you might choose to take a break during the day. You can close the door to your office or go into your bedroom at home for 10 minutes to relax. Use the time to breathe deeply, do the visualizations, or meditate. You will be much calmer and more relaxed afterward.

Physical Exercise

Women with anxiety symptoms should do moderate exercise on a regular basis, at least three times a week. Aerobic exercise can help improve circulation and oxygenation, thereby providing a relaxing effect. It is important, however, to do your exercise routine in a slow, comfortable manner, so as not to intensify your symptoms. Frenetic exercise that is too fast-paced is unhealthy if you are already nervous and tense; it can actually stress and exhaust you further. Pick a tempo that feels relaxing and comfortable.

To do the yoga stretches and acupressure massage described in this book, I recommend that you set aside a half-hour each day for the first week or two of starting your self help program. Try all the exercises. After an initial period of exploration, choose the ones that you enjoy the most and that seem to give you the most relief. Practice them on a regular basis so they can help prevent and reduce your symptoms.

Conclusion

I wish to reaffirm that each of us can do a tremendous amount for herself to assure optimal health and well-being. By having access to information, education, and health resources, every woman can play a major role in creating her own state of good health. Practice the beneficial self help techniques that I've outlined in this book. Follow good nutritional habits, exercise, and practice regular stress-reduction techniques. By combining good principles of self-care along with your regular medical care, you can enjoy the same wonderful results that my patients and I have had for a life of good health and well-being.

Bibliography

Chapter 3, Articles

Abraham, G. E. Nutritional factors in the etiology of the premenstrual syndrome. *Journal of Reproductive Medicine* 1983; 28:446–64.

Boulenger, J. P., et al. Increased sensitivity to caffeine in patients with panic disorders: Preliminary evidence. *Archives of General Psychiatry* 1984; 41:1067–71.

Bruce, M. Anxiogenic effects of caffeine in patients with anxiety disorders. *Archives of General Psychiatry* 1992; 49:867-9.

Bruce, M., and M. Lader. Caffeine abstention in the management of anxiety disorders. *Psychological Medicine* 1989; 19:211–14.

Charney, D. S., et al. Increased anxiogenic effects of caffeine in panic disorders. *Archives of General Psychiatry* 1985; 42:233–43.

Chou, Tony. Wake up and smell the coffee: caffeine, coffee and the medical consequences. *The Western Journal of Medicine* 1992; 157(5):544-53.

Christensen, L. Psychological distress and diet—effects of sucrose and caffeine. *Journal of Applied Nutrition* 1988; 40(1):44–50.

Dalton, K. Diet of women with severe premenstrual syndrome and the effect of changing to a three-hourly starch diet. *Stress Medicine* 1992; 8:544-53.

Dalvit-McPhillips, S. A dietary approach to bulimia treatment. *Physiology and Behavior* 1984; 33(5):769–75.

Freund, G. Benzodiazepine receptor loss in brains of mice after chronic alcohol consumption. *Life Sciences* 1980; 27(11):987–92.

Fullerton, D. T., et al. Sugar, opioids and binge eating. *Brain Research Bulletin* 1985; 14(6):673–80.

Goei, G. S., et al. Dietary patterns of patients with premenstrual tension. *Journal of Applied Nutrition* 1982; 34(1):4–11.

Heishman, S. and J. Henningfield. Stimulus functions in humans: the relation to dependence potential. *Neuroscience and Behavioral Reviews* 1992; 16:273-287.

Jones, D. V. Influence of dietary fat on self-reported menstrual symptoms. *Physiology and Behavior* 1987; 40(4):483–87.

King, D. S. Can allergic exposure provoke psychological symptoms? A double-blind test. *Biological Psychiatry* 1981; 16(1):3–19.

Manu, P., et al. Food intolerance in patients with chronic fatigue. *International Journal of Eating Disorders* 1993; 13(2):203-9.

Lee, M. A., et al. Anxiety and caffeine consumption in people with anxiety disorders. *Psychiatry Research* 1985; 15:211–17.

Lee, M. A., et al. Anxiogenic effects of caffeine on panic and depressed patients. *American Journal of Psychiatry* 1988; 145(5):632–35.

Levy, M., and E. Zylber-Katz. Caffeine metabolism and coffee-attributed sleep disturbances. *Clinical Pharmacology and Therapeutics* 1983; 33(6):770–75.

Monteiro, M. G., et al. Subjective feelings of anxiety in young men after ethanol and diazepam infusions. *Journal of Clinical Psychiatry* 1990; 51(1):12–16.

Rainey, J. M., Jr., et al. Specificity of lactate infusion as a model of anxiety. *Psychopharmacology Bulletin* 1984; 20(1):45–9.

Rogers, S. Chemical sensitivity: breaking the paralyzing paradigm. *Internal Medicine World Report* 1992; 7(3)1.15-16.

Rossignol, A. M. Caffeine-containing beverages and premenstrual syndrome in young women. *American Journal of Public Health* 1985; 75(11):1335–37.

Rossignol, A. M., et al. Tea and premenstrual syndrome in the People's Republic of China. *American Journal of Public Health* 1989; 79(1):67–69.

Rossignol, A.M. Do women with PMS self-medicate with caffeine? *Epdemiology* 1991; 2(6):403-8.

Rossignol, A. M., and H. Bonnlander. Caffeine-containing beverages, total fluid consumption, and premenstrual syndrome. *American Journal of Public Health* 1990; 80(9):1106–10.

Sanders, L. R., et al. Refined carbohydrate as a contributing factor in reactive hypoglycemia. *Southern Medical Journal* 1982; 75:1072.

Shirlow, M. J., and C. D. Mathers. A study of caffeine consumption and symptoms: indigestion, palpitations, tremor, headache, and insomnia. *International Journal of Epidemiology* 1985; 14(2):239–48.

Chapter 5, Books

Castleman, M. *The Healing Herbs*. Emmaus, PA: Rodale Press, 1991.

Crook, W., M.D. *Chronic Fatigue Syndrome and the Yeast Connection*. Jackson, TN: Professional Books, 1992.

Crook, W., M.D. *The Yeast Connection*. Jackson, TN: Professional Books, 1983.

Erasmus, U. *Fats and Oils*. Burnaby, BC, Canada: Alive Books, 1986.

Gittleman, A. L. *Supernutrition for Women*. New York: Bantam Books, 1991.

Hasslering, B., S. Greenwood, M.D., and M. Castleman. *The Medical Self-Care Book of Women's Health*. New York: Doubleday, 1987.

Hogladaroom, G., R. McCorkle, and N. Woods. *The Complete Book of Women's Health*. Englewood Cliffs, NJ: Prentice-Hall, 1982.

Kirschmann, J., and L. Dunne. *Nutrition Almanac*. New York: McGraw-Hill, 1984.

Lambert-Lagace, L. *The Nutrition Challenge for Women*. Palo Alto, CA: Bull Publishing, 1990.

Lark, S., M.D. *Heavy Menstrual Flow and Anemia Self Help Book*. Berkeley, CA: Celestial Arts, 1996.

Lark, S., M.D. *Chronic Fatigue and Tiredness Self Help Book*. Berkeley, CA: Celestial Arts, 1995.

Lark, S., M.D. *Fibroid Tumors and Endometriosis Self Help Book*. Berkeley, CA: Celestial Arts, 1995.

Lark, S., M.D. *Menopause Self Help Book*. Berkeley, CA: Celestial Arts, 1990.

Lark, S., M.D. *Menstrual Cramps Self Help Book*. Berkeley, CA: Celestial Arts, 1995.

Lark, S., M.D. *Premenstrual Syndrome Self Help Book*. Berkeley, CA: Celestial Arts, 1984.

Mowrey, D., Ph.D. *The Scientific Validation of Herbal Medicine*. New Canaan, CT: Keats Publishing, 1986.

Murray, M., N.D. *The 21st Century Herbal*. Bellevue, WA: Vita-Line, Inc., 1992.

Padus, E. *The Woman's Encyclopedia of Health and Natural Healing*. Emmaus, PA: Rodale Press, 1981.

Reuben, C., and J. Priestly, M.D. *Essential Supplements for Women*. New York: Perigree Books, 1988.

Trowbridge, J., M.D., and M. Walker, D.M.P. *The Yeast Syndrome*. New York: Bantam Books, 1988.

Chapter 5, Articles

Abbey, L. C. Agoraphobia. *Journal of Orthomolecular Psychiatry* 1982; 11:243–59.

Abraham, G. E. Magnesium deficiency in premenstrual tension. *Magnesium Bulletin* 1982; 1:68–73.

Abraham, G. E., and J. T. Hargrove. Effect of vitamin B_6 on premenstrual symptomatology in women with premenstrual tension syndrome: A double-blind cross-over study. *Infertility* 1980; 3:155–65.

Andersen, R. A. Chromium, diabetes mellitus and lipid metabolism. *Journal of the American College of Nutrition* 1992; 11(5):607.

Andersen, R. A., et al. Chromium supplementation of humans with hypoglycemia. *Federation Proceeding* 1984; 43:471.

Baranov, A. I. Medicinal uses of ginseng and related plants in the Soviet Union: Recent trends in the Soviet literature. *Journal of Ethnopharmacology* 1982; 6:339–53.

Boman, B. L-tryptophan: a rational anti-depressant and a natural hypnotic? *Australian and New Zealand Journal of Psychiatry* 1988; 22(1):83–97.

Bordoni, A., et al. Treatment of premenstrual syndrome with essential fatty acids (evening primrose oil). *Journal of Clinical Medicine* 1987; 68(1):23.

Brush, M. G., and M. Perry. Pyridoxine and the premenstrual syndrome. *Lancet* 1985; 1:1339.

Buist, R. A. Anxiety neurosis: The lactate connection. *International Clinical Nutrition Review* 1985; 5:1–4.

Carlson, R. J. Longitudinal observations of two cases of organic anxiety syndrome. *Psychosomatics* 1986; 27(7):529–31.

Cheraskin, E., et al. Daily vitamin C consumption and fatigability. *Journal of the American Geriatric Society* 1976; 24(3):136–37.

Chow, B. F., and H. F. Stone. The relationship of vitamin B_{12} to carbohydrate metabolism and diabetes mellitus. *The American Journal of Clinical Nutrition* 1957; 5:431.

Elghamry, M. I., and I. M. Shihata. Biological activity of phytoestrogens. *Planta Medica* 1965; 13:352–57.

Facchinetti, F. Oral magnesium successfully relieves premenstrual mood changes. *Obstetrics and Gynecology* 1991; 78(2):177–181.

Fitten, L. J., et al. L-tryptophan as a hypnotic in special patients. *Journal of the American Geriatric Society* 1985; 33:294.

Formica, P. E. The housewife syndrome. Treatment with the potassium and magnesium salts of aspartic acid. *Current Therapeutic Research* 1962; 4:98.

Gaby, A. R. Aspartic acid salts and fatigue. *Current Nutritional Therapeutics* November 1982.

Glen, I., et al. The role of essential fatty acids in alcohol dependence and tissue damage. *Alcoholism* (NY) 1987; 11(1):37.

Havsteen, B. Flavonoids, a class of natural products of high pharmacological potency. *Biochemical Pharmacology* 1983; 32:1141–48.

Horrobin, D. F. The role of essential fatty acids and prostaglandins in the premenstrual syndrome. *Journal of Reproductive Medicine* 1983; 28(7):465.

Kofle, K. H. Magnesium in psychotherapy. *Magnesium Research* 1988; 1(1):99.

Kuhnau, J. The flavonoids: A class of semi-essential food components: Their role in human nutrition. *World Review of Nutrition and Diet* 1976; 24:117–91.

Larsson, B., et al. Evening primrose oil in the treatment of premenstrual syndrome: A pilot study. *Current Therapeutic Research* 1989; 46:58.

Leathwood, P. D., et al. Aqueous extract of valerian root (Valeriana officinalis L.) improves sleep quality in man. *Pharmacology, Biochemistry, and Behavior* 1982; 17(1):65–71.

Lindahl, O., and L. Lindwall. Double blind study of valerian preparation. *Pharmacology, Biochemistry, and Behavior* 1989; 32(4):1065–66.

London, R. S. The effect of a nutritional supplement on premenstrual symptomatology. *Journal of the American College of Nutrition* 1991; 10(5):494–499.

London, R. S., et al. The effect of alpha-tocopherol on premenstrual symptomatology: A double-blind trial. *Journal of the American College of Nutrition* 1983; 2:115–22.

Mamalakis, G. Type A behavior and tissue linoleic acid: implications for stress management. *Journal of the American Collage of Nutrition* 1991; 11(5):606.

Middleton, E. The flavonoids. *Trends in Pharmaceutical Science* 1984; 5:335–38.

Mira, M., et al. Vitamin and trace element status of women with disordered eating. *American Journal of Clinical Nutrition* 1989; 50:940–44.

Mohler, H., et al. Nicotinamide is a brain constituent with benzodiazepine-like actions. *Nature* 1979; 278:563.

Nader, S. Premenstrual syndrome: tailoring treatment to symptoms. *Postgraduate Medicine* 1990; 90(1):173–180.

Neuringer, M., and W. E. Connor. Omega-3 fatty acids in the brain and retina: Evidence for their essentiality. *Nutrition Revue* 1986; 44(9):285.

Penland, J. Effects of trace element nutrition on sleep patterns in adult women. *Federation of the American Society of Experimental Biology* 1988; 2:A434.

Penland, J., and P. E. Johnnson. The dietary calcium and manganese effects on menstrual cycle symptoms. *American Journal of Obstetrics and Gynechology* 1993; 168(5):1417-23.

Puolakka, J., et al. Biochemical and clinical effects of treating the premenstrual syndrome with prostaglandin synthesis precursors. *Journal of Reproductive Medicine* 1985; 39(3):149–53.

Replogle, W. H., and F. J. Eicke. Megavitamin therapy in the reduction of anxiety and depression among alcoholics. *Journal of Orthomolecular Medicine* 1989; 4(4):221–24.

Rogers, S. Chemical sensitivity: breaking the paralyzing paradigm: how knowledge of chemical sensitivity enhances the treatment of chronic disease. *Internal Medicine World Report* 1992; 7(8):13–41.

Rosen, H., et al. Effects of the potassium and magnesium salts of aspartic acid on metabolic exhaustion. *Journal of Pharmaceutical Science* 1962; 51:592.

Rudin, D. O. The major psychoses and neuroses as omega-3 essential fatty acid deficiency syndrome: Substrate pellagra. *Biological Psychiatry* 1981; 16(9): 837–50.

Schneider-Helmert, D., and C. L. Spinweber. Evaluation of L-tryptophan for treatment of insomnia: A review. *Psychopharmacology* (Berlin) 1986; 89(1):1–7.

Shute, E. V. Notes on the menopause. *Canadian Medical Association Journal* 1937; 10:350.

Simpson, L. O. The etiopathogenesis of premenstrual syndrome as a consequence of altered blood rheology: A new hypothesis (evening primrose oil, fish oils). *Medical Hypotheses* 1988; 25(4):189.

Chapter 6, Books

Benson, R., and M. Klipper. *Relaxation Response*. New York: Avon, 1976.

Bourne, E. J. *The Anxiety and Phobia Workbook*. Oakland, CA: New Harbinger Publications, 1990.

Brennan, B. A. *Hands of Light*. New York: Bantam, 1987.

Davis, M. M., M. Eshelman, and E. Eshelman. *The Relaxation and Stress Reduction Workbook*. Oakland, CA: New Harbinger Publications, 1982.

Gawain, S. *Creative Visualization*. San Rafael, CA: New World Publishing, 1978.

Gawain, S. *Living in the Light*. Mill Valley, CA: Whatever Publishing, 1986.

Kripalu Center for Holistic Health. *The Self-Health Guide*. Lenox, MA: Kripalu Publications, 1980.

Loehr, J., and J. Migdow. *Take a Deep Breath*. New York: Villard Books, 1986.

Miller, E. *Self-Imagery*. Berkeley, CA: Celestial Arts, 1986.

Ornstein, R., and D. Sobel. *Healthy Pleasures*. Reading, MA: Addison-Wesley, 1989.

Padis, E. *Your Emotions and Your Health*. Emmaus, PA: Rodale Press, 1986.

Chapter 8, Books

Bailey, C. *Fit or Fat?* Boston: Houghton Mifflin, 1977.

Caillet, R., M.D., and C. Gross. *The Rejuvenation Strategy.* New York: Pocket Books, 1987.

Hanna, T. *Somatics.* Reading, MA: Addison-Wesley, 1988.

Huang, C. A. *Tai Ji.* Berkeley, CA: Celestial Arts, 1989.

Jerome, J. *Staying Supple.* New York: Bantam Books, 1987.

Kripalu Center for Holistic Health. *The Self-Help Guide.* Lenox, MA: Kripalu Publications, 1980.

McLish, R., and J. Vedral, Ph.D. *Perfect Parts.* New York: Warner Books, 1987.

Pinkney, C. *Callanetics: 10 Years Younger in 10 Hours.* New York: Avon, 1984.

Solveborn, S. A., M.D. *The Book About Stretching.* New York: Japan Publications, 1985.

Tobias, M., and M. Stewart. *Stretch and Relax.* Tucson, AZ: The Body Press, 1985.

Chapter 9, Books

Bell, L., and E. Seyfer. *Gentle Yoga.* Berkeley, CA: Celestial Arts, 1987.

Couch, J., and N. Weaver. *Runner's World Yoga Book.* New York: Runner's World Books, 1979.

Folan, L. *Lilias, Yoga, and Your Life.* New York: Macmillan, 1981.

Mittleman, R. *Yoga 28 Day Exercise Plan.* New York: Workman, 1969.

Iyengar, B. K. S. *Light on Yoga.* New York: Schocken Books, 1966.

Moore, M., and M. Douglas. *Yoga.* Arcane, ME: Arcane Publications, 1967.

Singh, R. *Kundalini Yoga.* New York: White Lion Press, 1988.

Chapter 10, Books

The Academy of Traditional Chinese Medicine. *An Outline of Chinese Acupuncture.* New York: Pergamon Press, 1975.

Bauer, C. *Acupressure for Women.* Freedom, CA: The Crossing Press, 1987.

Chang, S. *The Complete Book of Acupuncture.* Berkeley, CA: Celestial Arts, 1976.

Gach, M. R., and C. Marco. *Acu-Yoga.* Tokyo: Japan Publications, 1981.

Houston, F. M. *The Healing Benefits of Acupressure.* New Canaan, CT: Keats Publishing, 1974.

Kenyon, J. *Acupressure Techniques.* Rochester, VT: Healing Arts Press, 1980.

Nickel, D. J. *Acupressure for Athletes.* New York: Henry Holt, 1984.

Pendleton, B., and B. Mehling. *Relax With Self-Therap/Ease.* Englewood Cliffs, NJ: Prentice-Hall, 1984.

Teeguarden, I. *Acupressure Way of Health: Jin Shin Do.* Tokyo: Japan Publications, 1978.

Index

Binge eating, 82, 133, 145, 188, 190, 191, 242

Bioflavonoids, 92, 131–32, 140–41

Birth control pills, 21, 83, 129, 249

Bleeding, irregular, 21, 22

Bloating
    causes of, 86, 88, 89
    reducing, 91, 92–93, 135, 142, 193

Blood circulation
    exercises for, 196, 201, 204–05, 207–11, 219–20
    herbs for, 139, 144

Blood pressure
    high, 86, 87, 89
    lowering, 136, 161–62, 175, 246

Blood sugar level, 25–26, 81–82, 100
    diet and, 93, 94, 98–99, 101, 108
    physical exercise and, 192–93
    supplements for, 136, 137, 143–44, 145
    See also Hypoglycemia

Boat pose, 210–11

Bowel. See Intestinal distress

Bow (yoga exercise), 214–15

Brain function, 15, 189–90, 194
            See also Concentrating; Mind

Bread, whole grain, 102, 103

Breakfast meal plans, 99–103, 114–16

Breast tenderness, 132, 133

Breathing
    acupressure for, 221–22, 227–28, 232–34
    exercises, 162, 177–85, 215–17, 259
    problems with, 1, 11, 12, 28, 29, 178, 188, 189
    slowing, 162, 170, 177–85, 201, 259

Broccoli, 91, 107

Brown rice. See Rice

Buckwheat, 88, 90, 94, 101, 113, 131

BuSpar (buspirone hydrochloride), 247–48

Butter, substitutes, 102–03, 109, 124, 126, 146. See also Dairy products

Caffeine
    avoiding, 23, 29, 78–80, 82
    substitutes, 100, 121, 126, 237

Calcium
    nutrition of, 91, 105, 135–36
    sources of, 86–87, 95, 102, 121, 123, 136, 156

Calendar, 33–57

Cancer, 86, 87, 107

Candida, 82, 84, 88, 143

Carbohydrates, 81, 93, 94, 101, 104, 108

Cardiovascular system. See Blood circulation; Heart

Carob, 121, 126

Carrots, 91, 105, 108

Casseroles, 110, 113, 124–25

Cauliflower, 91, 105, 107

Centering, 162–64, 179–80

Cereals, 101–02, 103, 115, 116

Cheese, 86, 89, 123. See also Dairy products

Chest pain/tension, 12, 29, 227–28

Chicken. See Poultry

Children, anxiety and, 16, 17, 21, 168–69

Child's pose, 203

Chlordiazepoxide hydrochloride, 242

Chocolate, 27, 78–79, 80, 121, 126, 237. See also Caffeine

Cholesterol, 136, 137, 145–46

Chromium, 136–37

Clonazepam, 242

Clorazepate, 242

Cobra pose, 208–10

Coffee, 29, 78–80, 100, 121, 126, 135. See also Caffeine

Color breathing, 180–81, 182–83

Color visualizations, 169–71

Concentrating
    difficulty in, 11, 82, 100, 193
    improving, 162–64, 179–80, 190, 193
    See also Brain function; Mind

Condiments, 81, 89

Constipation. See Intestinal distress

Copper, 94

Corn, 88–89, 90, 94, 95, 102

Cortisol, 24, 26, 82

Cortisone, 9, 188

Counseling, 2, 160, 244. See also Psychotherapy

Crackers, 102

Cramps
    diet and, 87, 92, 93–94
    relieving, 203–04, 229–32
    supplements for, 92, 93–94, 129, 135, 145

Cravings. See Nutrition, cravings

Dairy products, 85–87, 100, 102, 115, 123–24, 126

Dalmane, 243

Deep breathing, 178

Depression, 11, 26, 27, 131, 184
    diet and, 86, 87, 88, 93
    drugs for, 191–92, 244–46, 247, 251
    exercises for, 172, 173–74, 183–84, 191–92, 232–34
    menopause and, 22, 184, 191, 251
    menstrual cycle and, 18, 184, 191, 232–34
    supplements for, 91, 139–40, 144, 148–49
    See also Mood swings

Desipramine, 244

Desserts, 25, 27, 81, 83, 93

Desyrel, 245–46

Diagnosis, 4, 11, 12, 24

Diarrhea. See Intestinal distress

Diazepam. See Valium

Dietary principles. *See* Nutrition

Digestion

exercises for, 201, 214–15, 229, 237

foods that ease, 92, 93, 94, 104, 108, 109

foods that hinder, 86, 87, 88, 94, 95, 96, 106

supplements for, 127, 136, 137, 139, 142–43, 144, 147

Dinner, 104–13, 114, 117–19

Dizziness, 12, 25, 27, 193

Dollar pose, 206–07

Doxepin, 244

Drugs, 239–55

addiction to, 2, 188, 191, 193, 196, 240, 243

antidepressants, 2, 21, 191–92, 244–46

for anxiety, 2, 239–48

appropriate use of, 2, 239–41

benzodiazepines, 242–44

beta-blockers, 29, 246–47

BuSpar (buspirone hydrochloride), 247–48

for depression, 191–92, 244–46, 247, 251

for hyperthyroidism, 247, 252–54, 255

for menopause, 23, 240, 242, 244, 250–52, 255

for mitral valve prolapse, 29

physical exercise vs., 191–92

for PMS, 21, 242, 244, 248–50, 255

See also Birth control pills; Hormonal replacement therapy

Eating habits. *See* Nutrition

Elavil, 244

Emotions, 72–73, 78, 97

exercises for, 181, 196–97, 202, 203–04, 211–12, 219, 237

See also Anxiety; Depression; Fear; Mood swings

Endocrine system

anxiety and, 10, 18–26

exercises for, 169, 170, 171, 182–83, 201, 221–22

stress and, 73, 182–83, 187–88

See also Adrenal glands

Energizing techniques

acupressure, 223–25, 229, 232–34

breathing exercises, 178, 183–84

color visualizations, 170–72

dietary, 87, 91, 92, 93, 124, 134

herbal, 139–40, 142, 143, 144

hormonal replacement therapy, 251

physical exercise, 189

vitamins and minerals, 92–93, 128, 130, 131, 133–34

yoga, 204–05, 211–15

See also Fatigue

Erasing stress, 166–68

Essential fatty acids. *See* Fatty acids

Estrace, 252

Estradiol, 251–52

Estrogen

anxiety and, 19–20, 128–29, 248–49

diet and, 83, 95, 131–32, 140–42

herbs and, 140–42, 144

liver and, 19–20, 128–29

menopause and, 22–23, 132, 251

phytoestrogens and, 131–32, 140–42, 144

PMS and, 19–20, 141, 251

Estrogen replacement therapy, 23, 83, 129, 132, 141, 240, 249, 250–52

Estrone, 251–52

Estropipate, 252

Exercises

acupressure, 219–37, 260

breathing, 162, 177–85, 215–17, 259

physical. *See* Physical exercise

relaxation. *See* Relaxation techniques

yoga, 196, 201–17, 260

Eyes, 24, 203–04

Face, swelling of, 203–04

Familial predisposition, 15–16

Fast food, 89, 98

Fatigue, 25, 160, 164

chronic, 11, 133–34, 139–40, 144, 170

diet and, 79, 82, 86, 87, 88, 95, 100, 110

energizing techniques. *See* Energizing techniques

medical disorders causing, 23, 26, 27, 29, 86, 131

menopause and, 22–23, 251

menstrual cycle and, 18, 19, 20, 21, 93, 131

Fats, 20, 86, 96, 99, 104, 106

Fatty acids, 95–96, 129, 133, 137, 145–47, 155

Fear, 1, 11, 12, 159, 166–69. *See also* Phobias

Feet, symptoms in, 9, 11, 12

Fiber, 93, 94, 101, 125

Fight-or-flight response, 8–9, 11, 12, 79, 160, 185–86

Fish, 90, 96, 106, 109–10, 113, 119, 145, 146–47

Flax, 95, 109, 115, 116, 124, 146

Flour, 81, 82, 94–95, 125, 126

Fluid retention, 86, 89, 91, 191

Fluoxetine hydrochloride, 245–46

Flurazepam, 243

Focusing, 162–64, 179–80

Food. *See* Nutrition

Food additives, 82, 85, 89

Food allergies, 11, 27–28, 77, 86, 91–92, 95, 99

foods to avoid, 27, 84, 85, 86, 88, 95

herbs for, 139–40, 142–44

Fruit, 61, 81, 90, 92–93, 99, 101, 131, 141

Fruit juices, 93, 100, 101

Gamma amino butyric acid (GABA), 15
Gamma linolenic acid (GLA), 129, 133,
    145–46
Gas. See Intestinal distress
Genetics, 15–16
Ginger, 121, 139, 142–43
Glandular breathing, 183
Glandular system. See Endocrine
    system
Glucose metabolism, 25–26, 81–82, 128,
    134, 136, 137
Gluten, avoiding, 88–89, 95
Grain beverages, 100, 121, 123, 126
Grains. See Whole grains
Greens, 87, 91, 105, 107
Grounding techniques, 162–64, 179–80

Halcion, 243
Half-wheel pose, 215–17
Hands, symptoms in, 9, 11, 12, 24
Headaches, 27, 129, 133, 142, 246
    exercises for, 206–07, 208–10,
        215–17, 221–22
Heart
    anxiety and stress and, 1, 10, 29, 73
    fats and, 86, 87, 106
    palpitations of, 12, 25, 29, 246
    strengthening, 135, 136, 140,
        188–89, 194, 196
    See also Mitral valve prolapse
Heart disease, 86, 87, 106, 135
Heart rate
    for aerobic exercise, 198
    lowering, 161–62, 170, 175, 187, 201,
        246
    nervous system control of, 8–9
    rapid, 1, 11, 12, 23, 28, 29, 189
Herbs, 137–44
    for anxiety, 138–39, 144

benefits of, 137–38
for chronic fatigue and depression,
    139–40, 144
for flavoring, 111, 125, 126
for food allergies and hypoglycemia,
    142–45
formulas, 149, 151, 152
how to use, 147
for menopause and PMS, 23, 139,
    140–42, 144, 152
teas, 80, 100, 114, 121, 139
Home life, stress and, 70–71
Honey, 83, 122, 126
Hormonal replacement therapy, 21, 23,
    83, 129, 132, 141, 240, 248–52
Hormones, 19–20, 22–23, 95, 124, 131.
    See also Adrenal glands; Endocrine
    system; Estrogen; Progesterone;
    Prostaglandins
Hot flashes, 21, 22, 79, 132, 141
    treatment of, 140, 221–22, 232–34, 240,
        251
Hummus, 106, 118
Hydrotherapy, 174–75
Hyperthyroidism, 2, 11, 23–25, 252
    endocrine glands and, 24–25, 182–83,
        187–88
    treatment of, 150–51, 194, 224, 247,
        252–54, 255
    See also Thyroid gland
Hypoglycemia, 25–26
    diet and, 25, 26, 77, 82, 83, 84, 99
    emotions and, 2, 25, 26, 184
    endocrine glands and, 182–83, 187–88
    exercises for, 183–84, 193–94, 195,
        221–25, 227–28
    supplements for, 26, 139–40, 142–44,
        150–51

Illness, stress and, 17, 69. See also
    Immune system

Imipramine, 244
Immune system
    anxiety and stress and, 10, 26–28,
        73, 183
    diet and, 87, 88, 91, 127, 130, 136
    exercises for, 169, 182–83, 201,
        215–17, 223–25
    herbs for, 140, 143
Inderal, 246–47
Indigestion. See Digestion
Inflammation, 87, 92
Inner child, healing the, 168–69
Insomnia
    causes of, 11, 23, 191
    devices for, 175
    drugs for, 243, 251
    exercises for, 191–92, 196, 206–07,
        221–22, 226–27
    menopause and, 22, 132, 138, 141,
        243, 251
    supplements for, 129–30, 134, 135,
        138–39, 141, 144
Insulin, 25, 26, 81–82, 136, 137
Intestinal distress
    causes of, 12, 23, 87, 88, 94, 129
    constipation, 142–43, 193
    diarrhea, 134, 135, 142–43
    gas, 88, 94, 139
    irritable bowel syndrome, 87,
        129, 242
    relieving, 93, 94, 101, 134, 193, 201,
        212–13
    supplements for, 134, 135, 139,
        142–43
    See also Fiber
Iodine, 96, 254
Iron, 79, 94, 105, 107
Irritability, 11, 20, 25, 26, 190, 249
    diet and, 78–79, 82, 100, 133, 135
    drugs for, 249, 251
    exercises for, 170–71, 183–84, 203

Nervous system, 8–9, 79, 84, 170, 179
   exercises for, 169, 201, 214–15
   supplements for, 129, 135, 136,
     138–39
   See also Sympathetic nervous
     system
Nervous tension
   diet and, 82, 93, 94, 99, 100, 128–29,
     133, 135
   exercises for, 159–76, 206–07,
     208–10, 214–17, 221–25
   physical exercise and, 189, 190, 191,
     192, 196
   stress and, 69, 160
   See also Irritability
Night sweats, 132, 240
Norepinephrine, 79, 244–45
Norethindrone, 252
Norlutin, 252
Norpramin, 244
Nortriptyline, 244
Nut butters, 99, 102, 103
Nut milk, 87, 100, 123
Nutrition
   addiction to foods. See Addiction,
     to foods
   allergies. See Food allergies
   anxiety and stress and, 2, 62
   binge eating/overeating, 82, 133,
     145, 188, 190, 191, 242
   cravings, 21, 27, 82, 85, 132, 193,
     214, 237
   dietary principles, 77–96
   emotional attachment to food, 78, 97
   evaluating eating habits, 59–62
   fast food, 89, 98
   food additives, 82, 85, 89
   foods that help, 60–62, 90–96
   foods that stress, 20, 59–60, 78–90
   gradually changing habits, 97–98,
     258–59

junk food, 78, 89, 97, 98, 188
   meal plans, 97–103, 104–11, 114
   menus, 103, 111–13
   recipes, 114–26
   substituting healthy ingredients,
     120–26
   supplements, 127–52, 258–59
   See also Fatty acids; Herbs; Miner-
     als; Vitamins
Nuts, 21, 61, 95–96, 105, 129, 145

Oak tree meditation, 163
Oats, 88–89, 101–02
Ogen, 252
Oils, 62, 90, 95–96, 124, 132, 146–47
Osteoporosis, 24, 89, 135
Oxazepam, 242

Pancreas. See Insulin
Panic disorder, 8, 9, 11–12, 15
   drugs for, 240, 242, 244, 245, 247
   mitral valve prolapse and, 29,
     246–47
   physical exercise and, 64, 189, 192,
     197–98
   supplements for, 148–49
   See also Exercises; Nutrition
Pasta, 94–95, 113, 120
Peaceful, slow breathing, 179
Peas, 86, 91, 93–95, 105, 108–09, 117
Phobias, 12, 13–15, 189, 192, 197, 240.
     See also Agoraphobia; Fear
Physical exercise, 187–200, 259–60
   aerobic, 63, 187, 190, 195, 197,
     259–60
   benefits of, 187–93
   evaluating fitness, 63–67, 195–96
   motivating self for, 198–99
   over-exercise, 64
   self help program for, 63–67,
     195—200, 259–60

types of, 63, 197
Phytoestrogens, 131–32, 140–42, 144
Pituitary gland, 182–83, 221–22. See
     also Beta endorphins; Insulin
PMS (premenstrual syndrome), 18–22
   anxiety and mood swings and,
     18–21, 133, 141, 184, 190, 191,
     244, 248–49
   causes of, 19–22, 248–49
   diet and, 77, 79, 82, 83, 86, 87, 88, 95,
     108
   drugs for, 21, 242, 244, 248–50, 255
   endocrine glands and, 182–83,
     187–88
   exercises for, 182–84, 193, 203–04,
     212–13, 229–32
   fatigue and, 18, 19, 20, 21
   fatty acids for, 95, 145
   herbs for, 139, 140–42, 144
   hormones and, 19–20, 83, 131, 132,
     141, 248–50, 251
   insomnia and, 243
   minerals for, 133, 134, 150
   risk factors for, 21
   vitamins for, 93–94, 129, 131, 132,
     150
Potassium, 79, 89, 91, 134–35
   sources of, 91, 92–93, 95, 96, 101,
     108, 135, 140
Potatoes, 81, 91, 93, 107, 109, 124
Potato milk, 87, 100, 102, 123
Poultry, 87, 90, 96, 106, 109, 124–25
Premarin, 252
Premenstrual syndrome. See PMS
Progesterone, 19–20, 22–23, 95, 132,
     141–42, 248–50
Progestin therapy, 250–52
Propranolol hydrochloride, 246–47
Propylthiouracil, 253–54
Prostaglandins, 87, 95, 109, 129, 133,
     134, 145–46

About Susan M. Lark, M.D.

Susan M. Lark, M.D., is a noted authority on women's health care and preventative medicine. Dr. Lark has been on the clinical faculty of Stanford University Medical School, Division of Family and Community Medicine, where she continues to teach. She has been the director of a number of clinical programs for women and worked with thousands of patients in her twenty years of private practice. Dr. Lark lectures widely on women's health issues and is the author of a series of books published by Celestial Arts including: *PMS Self Help Book, The Menopause Self Help Book, Menstrual Cramps Self Help Book, Fibroid Tumors & Endometriosis Self Help Book, Heavy Menstrual Flow & Anemia Self Help Book, Anxiety & Stress Self Help Book, Chronic Fatigue Self Help Book, The Estrogen Decision Self Help Book,* and *The Women's Health Companion.* She also presents workshops and seminars on women's health issues. If you would like to contact her for more personalized guidance, Dr. Lark is available for personal or phone consultation at (415) 964-7268.

Acknowledgment

The author and publisher wish to extend a special acknowledgment to Shelly Reeves-Smith and Cracom Corporation for permission to reproduce the creative line drawings found in the food section of this book. These and additional drawings, together with a collection of wonderful recipes, may be found in the cookbook *Just a Matter of Thyme* available in your local gift or book store. Inquires may be addressed to Among Friends, P.O. Box 1476, Camdenton, MO 65020 or call toll free (800) 377-3566.

Dr. Susan Lark's
Complete Self Help Library on Women's Health

❧ Heavy Menstrual Flow & Anemia

One in five American women suffers from anemia due to iron or folic acid deficiency. Dr. Lark helps you understand and identify the causes, symptoms, and diagnosis of anemia, as well as heavy and irregular menstrual bleeding. Assess your symptoms and begin your own natural self help treatment. —*164 pages*

❧ Anxiety & Stress

Millions of women suffer from emotional distress, nervous tension, panic, and anxiety...often on a daily basis. Dr. Lark discusses the causes, symptoms, and diagnosis of anxiety and other emotional conditions, and guides you through an effective self help treatment program. —*284 pages*

❧ Chronic Fatigue

Chronic fatigue is one of the most common—and most commonly misunderstood—medical complaints for which women seek their doctors' advice. Dr. Lark has designed programs to help you relieve chronic fatigue syndrome, as well as underlying conditions, including candida, infections, depression, allergies, and fatigue due to PMS, menopause, and thyroid conditions. —*234 pages*

❧ Fibroid Tumors & Endometriosis

Over 40% of American women develop fibroid tumors of the uterus. Endometriosis is common to menstruating women from ages 20 to 45. Both conditions cause a variety of distressing symptoms. Identify the signs, symptoms, and risk factors, and then formulate your own treatment program with Dr. Lark's help. —*264 pages*

❧ Menstrual Cramps

Fifty percent of all women suffer from painful menstrual periods. Some have symptoms so severe that they are unable to cope with their normal daily activities. This valuable book describes types and causes of menstrual pain, helps women evaluate their own symptoms, and presents a comprehensive self help program. —*224 pages*

❧ The Estrogen Decision

Should you use estrogen during and after menopause? Get the facts on the benefits, side effects, and risks of estrogen, progesterone, and hormone replacement therapy (HRT). Dr. Lark discusses the latest information on the issues surrounding menopause, and offers alternative treatments for specific menopausal symptoms. —*316 pages*

❧ Menopause

You don't have to dread menopause. Dr. Lark offers the first completely safe, practical, all-natural master plan for relieving and preventing menopause symptoms including irritability and hot flashes...as well as a plan to help eliminate the long-term risk of osteoporosis and breast and uterine cancer. —*240 pages*

❧ Premenstrual Syndrome

Dr. Lark's plan helps you eliminate the causes of PMS symptoms, including anxiety, pain, weight gain, chocolate cravings, mood swings, depression, bloating, and breast tenderness. Learn how to deal with sugar cravings and caffeine addiction, prevent depression and mood swings, and alleviate pain. —*240 pages*

❧ The Women's Health Companion: Self Help Nutrition Guide and Cookbook

The only cookbook that answers women's special nutritional needs, including recipes to prevent and treat PMS, osteoporosis, breast cancer, heart disease, menopause, fibrocystic breast disease, and endometriosis. Also includes menus and a discussion of how to make an easy transition to your healthy new diet. —*370 pages*